Missing the Meaning?

Missing the Meaning?

A Cognitive Neuropsychological Study of the Processing of Words by an Aphasic Patient

David Howard
Sue Franklin

A Bradford Book
The MIT Press
Cambridge, Massachusetts
London, England

This book was set in Palatino by Asco Trade Typesetting Ltd., Hong Kong, and printed and bound by Halliday Lithograph in the United States of America.

Library of Congress Cataloging-in-Publication Data

Howard, David, 1951–
  Missing the meaning? : a cognitive neuropsychological study of the processing of words by an aphasic patient / David Howard, Sue Franklin.

      p.   cm.—(Issues in the biology of language and cognition)
  "A Bradford book."
  Bibliography: p.
  Includes indexes.
  ISBN 0-262-08178-4
  1. Aphasia—Case studies. 2. Neurolinguistics. I. Franklin, Sue. II. Title. III. Series.
  [DNLM: 1. Aphasia. 2. Cognition. 3. Neurophysiology. 4. Psycholinguistics.
WL 340.5 H848m]
RC425.H65   1988
616.85′52—dc 19
DNLM/DLC
for Library of Congress

88-13006
CIP

Contents

PART II
Interpretations and Implications

Series Foreword

The MIT Press series on Issues in the Biology of Language and Cognition brings new approaches, concepts, techniques, and results to bear on our understanding of the biological foundations of human cognitive capacities. The series will include theoretical, experimental, and clinical work that ranges from the basic neurosciences, clinical neuropsychology, and neuro-linguistics to formal modeling of biological systems. Studies in which the architecture of the mind is illuminated by both the fractionation of cognition after brain damage and formal theories of normal performance are specifically encouraged.

John C. Marshall

A Case Study in Neurolinguistics
John C. Marshall

Aphasiology—the study of acquired language disorders, their neuronal substrate, and implications for normal cognition—came of age in the closing decades of the nineteenth century. Triggered by Paul Broca's success in localizing "le souvenir du procédé qu'il faut suivre pour articuler les mots" (Broca, 1866), the discipline attracted scores of behavioral neurologists who, with Leibniz, saw language as a mirror of the mind. Across continental Europe (Charcot, 1883; Bianchi, 1886), the United Kingdom (Broadbent, 1884; Elder, 1897), and North America (Dercum, 1894; Gordinier, 1899), aphasic patients were compared, contrasted, and interpreted for the light that their deficits throw on the mental organ of language. But it was, above all, in the German-speaking lands that the fine art of detailed, extensive investigation of single cases was developed (see de Bleser, 1987).

At risk of encouraging cultural stereotypes, one could say that from Berlin to Breslau, and from Zurich to Prague (by way of Vienna), patients were documented with Prussian thoroughness and analyzed with teutonic precision. The result in this case was a thriving, progressive science. The combination of intensive behavioral investigation and explicit theory (as represented by the flow-charts first proposed in this context by Baginsky, 1871) was exactly what was required to found a rigorous neurolinguistics. The adequacy of the diagram-makers' models could be tested against the performance of each new, relevant patient who was seen, and the theory, where necessary, modified accordingly (see Morton, 1984).

When Europe destroyed itself in two world wars (and German ceased to be the universal language of science), much of this aphasiological tradition was lost. Henry Head (1926) reserved his bitterest scorn for Carl Wernicke and Ludwig Lichtheim, diagram-makers who, in Head's view would "lop and twist their cases to fit the procrustean bed of their hypothetical conceptions." For Head (as earlier for his intellectual mentor, John Hughlings Jackson), the goal was to describe what the patient could and could not do, without any theoretical preconceptions influencing the description. The extent to which the human mind is capable of such "virgin" observation is, of course, debatable. In Head's case, the result was a plethora of unorganized data that had little effect upon subsequent developments in aphasiology. In fairness, however, Head did collect a large range of observations from his patients; he could thus display, if not interpret or make theoretical sense of, the alarming variability that is seen between one aphasic patient and another.

The next mistake was to cover up this variability in the name of psychometrics and standardized test construction. No one could object to more stringent testing procedures and statistical analysis *per se*; but the "new objectivity" inevitably led to group studies (Weisenburg and McBride, 1935) in which all the interesting (and theoretically significant) differences between patients were swamped by measures of central tendency. Even when investigations explicitly attempted to isolate subgroups of aphasic patients (by factor-analysis, for example), the results were for the most part unrevealing—patients differ in overall severity and in which sensorimotor modality of language performance is most impaired (Schuell, Jenkins, and Jiménez-Pabón, 1964). Investigators simply lost sight of the fact that when an aphasia-battery is given to a large group of patients, the results are determined more by the nature of the test items than by the characteristics of the patients. Kurt Goldstein's motto—"Symptome sind ja nur Antworten auf unsere Fragen"—had been left behind in the Frankfurt Neurological Institute (Goldstein, 1923).

It was Norman Geschwind who, to his eternal credit, first revived the work of the German neurological tradition—or at least that part of the tradition that had been due to Wernicke and Liepmann (Geschwind, 1965). The problem, however, was that Geschwind's advocacy of the Wernicke-Lichtheim model of the aphasias was too persuasive: he convinced a substantial population of neurologists and neuropsychologists that the classical anatomoclinical theory was *true*. True, I emphasize, not merely a very fine attempt to understand the complexities of human language and its instantiation in the brain. Geschwind's own analyses of the inadequacies of classical theory (Geschwind, 1969) never attained the circulation enjoyed by the idea that there are seven (or eight) basic syndromes of aphasia and three syndromes of alexia. The Breslau-Boston classification (Goodglass and Kaplan, 1972) thus became "ground" rather than "figure." Patients would be "objectively" assigned to a particular taxonomic category (Broca's aphasia, Wernicke's aphasia, conduction aphasia ...) on the basis of their test performance. They then became available for group studies in which some further aspect of Broca's aphasia (Wernicke's aphasia ...) could be investigated.

What this research strategy overlooks is that, even after such subtyping, the groups are not homogeneous. As Benson (1979) writes, "Medical syndromes do not exist as fixed, consistent entities ... variability, inexactness and incompleteness are commonplace." A traditional aphasic syndrome is rather a set of family relationships, akin to Wittgenstein's analysis of the concept of a game (Marshall, 1982). Schwartz (1984) thus observes that "the category Broca's aphasia can be attributed no necessary feature, nor any combination of necessary features." If such a group is heterogeneous in terms of its defining characteristics, there are no good reasons to assume that all the members of the group will behave in the same fashion on any further test of cognitive performance.

Group studies based upon polytypic symptom-complexes are now widely (though not ubiquitously) regarded as invalid (Caramazza, 1984; Marshall and Newcombe, 1984). And have been superseded by ... exactly the kind of extensive single-case study that provided the driving force behind late-nineteenth-century attempts to understand the structure of cognition (Shallice, 1979). This new (or rather old) state of affairs has not been without critics who have asked how one can generalize from a sample of $n = 1$. The answer, of course, is that one cannot ... but also that science (as opposed to actuarial prediction) is not primarily in the business of generalizing from samples to populations. The explanatory power of science arises rather from theories that can account for whatever variability is observed in the world with as few principles as are necessary to attain descriptive adequacy (Chomsky, 1965).

The logic of the controversy is straightforward. Ellis (1987) characterizes the research program of taxonomic neuropsychology as follows:

> *Step One*: Study a patient (or set of patients) in order to give as precise a description as possible of their symptoms.
> *Step Two*: Assign the patient(s) to a syndrome category on the basis of the symptoms discovered in Step One.
> *Step Three*: Try to explain the *syndrome* in terms of impairment to one or more components of a theory of normal cognitive functioning.

The problems arise at step two. All polytypic syndromes fractionate (by definition and in point of fact); in a complex system, any individual symptom can be caused by a wide variety of different malfunctions. Mapping from step two to step three is accordingly liable to provoke more confusion than insight. The solution to the problems of step two "is both simple and straightforward—do away with it!" (Ellis, 1987). One should map the data from step one *directly* onto the cognitive theory of step three. No one individual patient with language disorder will suffice to erect a full theory of language functions (just as no one experiment with normal subjects answers all the questions). The performance of each patient is, however, either consistent with a particular theory, or not. If consistent (that is, interpretable in terms of available mechanisms), the theory is strengthened. If not, the theory must be modified (or jettisoned). And that's all there is to it! This "inherently progressive" (Shallice, 1979) aspect of cognitive neuropsychology was characteristic of the first golden age. The diagram-makers did not hesitate to revise their theories when counterevidence (from single-cases) was forthcoming. We could better honor their endeavors by following their research strategy than by reifying the diagrams in which they embodied *their* final theories.

Missing the meaning is a book that follows the spirit, not the letter, of the diagram-makers' achievements. David Howard and Sue Franklin describe *one* patient, MK, who, from the standpoint of taxonomic neurolinguistics, can be said to manifest *four* syndromes—Wernicke's aphasia, word deafness, surface dyslexia, and deep dysgraphia. Such a constellation of impairments could, of course, be quite fortuitous, analogous, for example, to a patient who had the misfortune to suffer simultaneously from toothache, appendicitis, influenza, and ingrowing toenails. On the other hand, it could be the case that the full range of overt symptomatology in different modalities of performance follows deductively from impairment to a small number of underlying components. If Howard and Franklin had terminated their investigation once the patient had been (multiply-) classified, we would have no way of resolving the issue. Accordingly, they take syndrome-assignment as a preliminary heuristic to help place the patient within existing domains of theory. But the real work starts, not stops, at this point.

On the basis of their best guess at the functional architecture of lexical processing, Howard and Franklin attempt to find theoretical coherence behind the superficially bewildering array of positive and negative symptoms. To achieve their goal, they must run multiple experiments on the patient, drawing upon many varied tests (and inventing others), and continuously changing their models to obtain maximal coverage of the data. This type of experimentation, which tests the examiner's ingenuity as much as the patient's capacity, is not easy, but it is the very core of current methodology.

In the development of modern case-study methodology, much attention was initially devoted to the discovery of "pure" syndromes. When it was realized that even the best-behaved of multisymptom syndromes was susceptible to fractionation, search turned to the elucidation of single-symptom "syndromes." Such cases, which do (with a little idealization!) exist, proved particularly pertinent to validating the existence of the routes and representations postulated by the new diagram-makers. They also forced minor modifications of existing models (usually the postulation of an additional box or arrow) when no extant route or representation could cover the observed pattern of performance.

By contrast, patients who showed multiple impairments across many different domains were often regarded as "too messy" to reveal a convincing functional architecture. Alternatively, those individual patients who did unambiguously manifest more than one "symptom-complex" were sometimes written up as if they were indeed separate patients. A well-known example is RG, a patient who presented with "phonological dyslexia," "surface dysgraphia," and "bilateral tactile aphasia" (Beauvois, Saillant, Meininger and Lhermitte, 1978; Beauvois and Derouesné, 1979; 1981). Lying behind this tendency to reify syndromes, there is a cautionary tale (Marshall and Newcombe, 1988) that Howard and Franklin have now spelled out in detail. *Missing the meaning* shows that these complex cases can be studied as individuals and that their performance, far from being messy, can be employed to drive significant advances in our understanding of neurolinguistic functions.

Missing the meaning, then, is an important book in at least three ways. First, it is an exemplary case study in its own right. Second, it demonstrates how theoretical insights can be obtained from individual patients with many superficially distinct language impairments. These insights are furthermore not available from "purer" cases, precisely because the interpretation of the former ("mixed") cases involves an intimate relationship between only apparently distinct symptoms. Last, but not least, *Missing the meaning* is a case study in how to pursue neurolinguistic inquiry. Lucidly written, with all the logical steps in the argument explicitly expressed, Howard and Franklin's book will, I hope, provide an ideal working introduction to the new cognitive neuropsychology.

References

Baginsky, A. 1871. "Aphasie in Folge schwerer Nierenerkrankungen." *Berliner Klinische Wochenschrift* 8: 428–431, 439–443.

Beauvois, M.-F., and Derouesné, J. 1979. "Phonological alexia: three dissociations." *Journal of Neurology, Neurosurgery and Psychiatry* 42: 1115–1124.

Beauvois, M.-F., and Derouesné, J. 1981. "Lexical or orthographic agraphia." *Brain* 104: 21–49.

Beauvois, M.-F., Saillant, B., Meininger, V., and Lhermitte, F. 1978. "Bilateral tactile aphasia: a tacto-verbal dysfunction." *Brain* 101: 381–401.

Benson, D. F. 1979. *Aphasia, Alexia, and Agraphia*. London: Churchill Livingstone.

Bianchi, L. 1886. "Un caso di sordite verbale." *Rivista Sperimentale di Freniatria* 12: 57–71.

Broadbent, W. H. 1884. "On a particular form of amnesia. Loss of nouns." *Medico-Chirurgical Transactions* 67: 249–264.

Broca, P. 1866. "Sur la faculté générale du langage, dans ses rapports avec la faculté du langage articulé." *Bulletin de la Societé d'Anthropologie*, Second Series 1: 377–382.

Caramazza, A. 1984. "The logic of neuropsychological research and the problem of patient classification in aphasia." *Brain and Language* 21: 9–20.

Charcot, J. M. 1883. "Des différentes formes de l'aphasie. 1. De la cécité verbale." *Progrès Médicale* (Paris) 11: 441–449.

Chomsky, N. 1965. *Aspects of the Theory of Syntax*. Cambridge, Mass.: MIT Press.

de Bleser, R. 1987. "From agrammatism to paragrammatism: German aphasiological traditions and grammatical disturbances." *Cognitive Neuropsychology* 4: 187–256.

Dercum, F. X. 1894. "A case of hemiplegia." *Journal of Nervous and Mental Disorders* 21: 609–613.

Elder, W. 1897. *Aphasia and the Cerebral Speech Mechanisms*. London: H. K. Lewis.

Ellis, A. W. 1987. "Intimations of modularity, or, the modelarity of mind: Doing cognitive neuropsychology without syndromes," in *The Cognitive Neuropsychology of Language*, M. Coltheart, G. Sartori, and R. Job, eds. London: Lawrence Erlbaum, 397–408.

Geschwind, N. 1965. "Disconnexion syndromes in animals and man." *Brain* 88: 237–294, 585–644.

Geschwind, N. 1969. "Problems in the anatomical understanding of the aphasias." in *Contributions to Clinical Neuropsychology*, A. L. Benton, ed. Chicago: Aldine, 107–128.

Goldstein, K. 1923. "Die Topik der Grosshirnrinde und ihrer klinischen Bedeutung." *Deutsche Zeitschrift für Nervenheilkunde* 77: 7–124.

Goodglass, H., and Kaplan, E. 1972. *The Assessment of Aphasia and Related Disorders*. Philadelphia: Lea and Febiger.

Gordinier, H. C. 1899. "A case of brain tumor at the base of the second frontal circonvolution." *American Journal of Medical Science* 117: 526–535.

Head, H. 1926. *Aphasia and Kindred Disorders of Speech*. Cambridge: Cambridge University Press.

Marshall, J. C. 1982. "What is a symptom-complex?" in *Neural Models of Language Processes*, M. A. Arbib, D. Caplan, and J. C. Marshall, eds. New York: Academic Press, 389–409.

Marshall, J. C., and Newcombe, F. 1984. "Putative problems and pure progress in neuropsychological single-case studies." *Journal of Clinical Neuropsychology* 6: 65–70.

Marshall, J. C., and Newcombe, F. 1988. "Parasyndromes and paragrammatism." *Aphasiology* 2: in press.

Morton, J. 1984. "Brain-based and non-brain-based models of language," in *Biological Perspectives on Language*, D. Caplan, A. R. Lecours, and A. Smith, eds. Cambridge, Mass.: MIT Press, 40–64.

Schuell, H., Jenkins, J. J., and Jiménez-Pabón, E. 1964. *Aphasia in Adults*. New York: Harper and Row.

Schwartz, M. 1984. "What the classical aphasia categories can't do for us, and why." *Brain and Language* 21: 3–8.

Shallice, T. 1979. "Case study approach in neuropsychological research." *Journal of Clinical Neuropsychology* 1: 183–211.

Weisenburg, T. H., and McBride, K. E. 1935. *Aphasia: a clinical and psychological study*. New York: Commonwealth Fund.

Acknowledgments

We have been working with MK now for several years. This book recounts only that segment of our results that deals with single word processing. A number of people have given us significant help. First we thank Dr. Ronald Zeegan for permission to study MK. Financial support was provided to Sue Franklin by North West Thames Regional Health Authority and, more recently, by the Medical Research Council. David Howard was supported by the Medical Research Council. Unpublished test materials have been made available by Sally Byng, Max Coltheart, Janice Kay, Karalyn Patterson, and Tim Shallice; we thank them. A large number of people have discussed issues related to MK with us; many of our early ideas were developed in conjunction with the London Single Case Study Group and we thank its members for their patient interest. We are particularly grateful to those who at various stages, have read and commented on this manuscript; we thank Rita Berndt, Brian Butterworth, Max Coltheart, Elaine Funnell, Stephen Monsell, and especially Karalyn Patterson. Our main thanks, though, go to MK and his wife Tylke for their cooperation and for the ways in which they have helped us over the years of these investigations.

Introduction

This book is devoted to the language performance of a single aphasic man. In one way he is not a particularly exceptional patient; his performance is close to the classical form of 'Wernicke's aphasia', a condition where, according to Goodglass and Geschwind (1976), "auditory comprehension is impaired, while fluency and ease of articulation are spared" (p. 418).

If giving the correct label to a patient's disorder were a complete analysis of the disorder, we would have little more to say. But it is our contention in this book that our patient MK has a number of quite selective, precise, and characterizable deficits that are responsible for his difficulties in single word processing. One of the purposes of this book is to show how MK's difficulties in processing single words can be accounted for in terms of a set of impairments to a model of word processing in normal people. In that sense this book is an example of 'the cognitive neuropsychological method' applied to the analysis of aphasic breakdown (see Coltheart 1984; Coltheart, Sartori and Job 1987; Shallice 1979a, 1988). We hope that the present study will exhibit some of the power of this approach and illustrate how an apparently bewildering array of features can be traced back to a relatively small number of impairments. We still feel excitement at the way this approach allows us to deal with the detailed patterns of our patients' problems.

While in terms of the syndrome labels of Goodglass, Geschwind, and their colleagues, MK is a fairly typical 'Wernicke's aphasic', in other ways he may be atypical. He demonstrates a number of types of breakdown that have not been very well described in the existing literature. Thus he shows a breakdown in auditory word comprehension that might be described as a kind of 'word deafness'. In reading words aloud, he makes errors that are characteristic of 'surface dyslexics', although, as we will argue, his pattern of surface dyslexia is qualitatively different from that of any other patient described so far. In writing words to dictation, MK makes semantic errors; indeed he shows all the features of 'deep dysgraphia'. In word repetition he also makes semantic errors; he shows the features of what Morton (1980b) described as "the auditory analogue of deep dyslexia." Our second aim in this book, then, is to provide detailed and comprehensive descriptions of

MK's performance in all these areas, some of which have been hitherto neglected in neuropsychological research. In doing this we devote the first section of the book to a review of the literature on these symptom-complexes, to bring together the relevant case descriptions in these areas. From this perspective, then, MK might be seen as four patients rolled into one.

We think that characterizing MK in terms of symptomcomplexes misses some important features of his performance. It misses the ways in which these patterns of breakdown are intimately related to each other. That they co-occur in the same patient is no accident; in MK's case they reflect the same set of underlying processing impairments. For example, we will argue that the same deficits that cause MK to make 'semantic errors in repetition' are also responsible for his 'deep dysgraphia'. Should one then simply abandon the notion of symptomcomplex? In the last section of the book we return to this issue; we argue that, where they are defined in the right way, symptomcomplexes are a useful conceptual tool in cognitive neuro-psychology. This is because they facilitate the comparison of patterns of performance across individual subjects. This leads us to a reexamination of the status of studies of single patients, in the light of our case study with MK. We argue that, where such studies are properly done, we can ensure that the results represent both a reliable portrait of MK's aphasia and that our conclusions can be generalized to include other patients and normal people.

Our third purpose in this book is to use our analysis of MK's impaired performance to draw conclusions about the nature of normal language performance. Any model of normal language that is sufficiently explicit will predict that certain kinds of breakdown can occur and other forms cannot. As Shallice (1979a) and Coltheart (1985) argue, cognitive neuropsycho-logical case studies can be used to provide evidence for or against particu-lar theories of normal processing. In the latter part of this book we will use our analysis of MK's performance to argue that some theoretical positions are not tenable, and we will draw some conclusions which we think could come only from neuropsychological evidence. In the main body of this book the analysis of MK's data will be in terms of an elaboration of Morton and Patterson's (1980) model of lexical processing, which in turn is derived from a succession of versions of Morton's 'logogen model' (see Morton 1964, 1970, 1979, etc). We use this model because it is the only one we know of that is sufficiently explicit and comprehensive to deal with all the single word processing tasks we used with MK. In the final section we will consider how some other theories might deal with some aspects of the data.

The first chapter of the book is a brief review of the relevant literature on the five symptomcomplexes which MK shows: Wernicke's aphasia, sur-face dyslexia, word deafness, semantic errors in repetition, and deep dysgraphia. The following chapters will consider his performance in a set of tasks in the following order: oral word reading, written word comprehension, spoken word comprehension, written and spoken naming, oral repetition and writing to dictation. This order has been chosen to maximize the probability of demonstrating how different symptoms relate to each other. Even so, we will occasionally need to retrace our steps, once the relevance of another question has been established. Using the classic method of cognitive neuropsychology, we examine the variables affecting performance in each of these tasks and the kinds of errors that MK makes. These results are interpreted in terms of a version of Morton and Patterson's (1980) model of lexical processing. In the final part of the book we summarize our conclusions about the elements in this model that are disrupted and impaired. Then we consider the implications our data have for accounts of lexical organization and reconsider the status of the five symptom-complexes and of the notion of symptomcomplexes in general. We end with a piece written by MK, which we feel conveys something of the consequences MK's aphasia has had for him.

There are three ways in which this book is concerned with the question of "Missing the meaning?" First, there is the question of whether describing MK's problems in terms of symptomcomplexes can capture the essential features of his performance. Second, we consider whether MK has lost some or all of his meaning representations for some words. And finally, we document how MK sometimes misses the correct meaning of a word he hears and instead accesses the semantics of another word closely related in sound; thus, he defined the word "cult" as "a little horse."

Chapter 1

Five Symptomcomplexes

1 Wernicke's aphasia

In 1874 Carl Wernicke provided the first clear description and theoretical interpretation of an aphasic patient who had a prominent deficit in word comprehension. This theoretical framework was developed further by Lichtheim (1885), and the approach was revived in the 1960s by Geschwind and his colleagues in Boston (US). This American school now uses the term 'Wernicke's aphasia' to describe a pattern of impairment that has, in their formulation, the following characteristics:

> In Wernicke's dysphasia, spontaneous speech is fluent, paraphasic and unmonitored, and auditory and written comprehension are poor. Performance in reading, writing and repetition parallels that of spontaneous speech. The patient is commonly unaware of his speech deficit and produces a flow of uncorrected, meaningless, well articulated sentences. (Albert, Goodglass, Helm, Rubens, and Alexander 1981, p. 76)

Wernicke had suggested that the deficit in word comprehension was primary; destruction of the "centre for acoustic word images" resulted in disordered paraphasic speech because of a failure in self-monitoring.

> Patients who do not comprehend the spoken word produce a seemingly confused type of speech with the result that they are often [...] regarded as mentally ill [...] Such a patient typically has many words at his command but often substitutes incorrect words for the correct expression. Repeated misspeaking, a characteristic of these patients, may prevail to such an extent that entire sentences are inserted at the wrong place, and slips of speech occur in the heat of the moment, resulting in complete distortion of meaning [...] One must postulate that the presence of the acoustic-imagery during speech production acts as a constant unconscious monitor, and that loss of such imagery results in a disruption of this monitoring process. (Wernicke and Friedlander 1883, pp. 170–171 in Eggert's translation)

In the earliest formulation, deficits in reading comprehension did not necessarily follow. Wernicke (1874) suggests that "the educated person" might have intact comprehension of written material, although oral reading would be disturbed in the same way as spontaneous speech production, again because of the failure in monitoring.

Lichtheim (1885), elaborating on Wernicke's system, suggests that there are three different types of sensory aphasia. He describes a patient who appeared absolutely deaf but who was able to hear the sound of a bell "even when it was rung most gently behind him" (p. 462). The patient showed no auditory comprehension, but speech production was not disturbed. Lichtheim interpreted this 'peripheral conduction speech deafness' as a disconnection of acoustic input from the center of auditory images. In this formulation, speech production is unimpaired because the auditory images are still able to exert their controlling, monitoring function on speech production. Wernicke (1885) subsequently suggested that 'subcortical sensory aphasia' would be a more appropriate term for this disorder.

The second type of sensory aphasia described by Lichtheim is due to destruction of the center for auditory word images. This results in the symptomcomplex that Wernicke had described—impaired comprehension and repetition, and fluent paraphasic speech production. The third type was named 'transcortical sensory aphasia' by Wernicke (1885). This is caused by disconnection of auditory word images from word concepts, resulting in severely disturbed comprehension. Repetition remains possible because the connection from auditory word images to motor word images remains intact; speech production is relatively intact although the patient may show some degree of paraphasia due to an inability to understand his or her own speech.

In their modern reformulation of the Wernicke-Lichtheim system, Albert et al. (1981) have described some features of the performance of Wernicke's aphasics in particular tasks. In speech production, there is an abundance of 'function words' (words from closed grammatical categories); and a wide variety of grammatical forms are used, but inappropriately. Word errors consist of both phonological and semantic paraphasias, as well as combinations of the two.

The auditory comprehension deficit is severe; the patient is often unable to point to items when they are named by the examiner. Sometimes, it is claimed, the patients may do better in following commands that involve movements of the whole body than in matching single words to pictures. According to a number of authors the auditory comprehension deficit is due to a difficulty in phonemic perception (e.g., Luria 1947; Goldstein 1948). The earliest proponent of this view was Wernicke himself: "there is a loss of word sound perception [...] the disorder is purely acoustic" (Wernicke 1906, pp. 226–7 in Eggert's translation). Thus Wernicke's aphasics may, for example, point to a picture of a 'tin' when told to point to the 'pin' (e.g., Gainotti, Caltagirone, and Ibba 1975; Baker, Blumstein, and Goodglass 1981). This view, however, has been challenged by other authors; Blumstein, Baker, and Goodglass (1977) found that errors in same/ different phoneme judgments were just as common among Broca's aphasics (whose comprehension is said to be good) as Wernicke's aphasics. In the light of this evidence, Albert et al. suggest that "the phonemic processing deficit in Wernicke's dysphasia is not at the perceptual or hearing level but at the level at which linguistic significance is associated with adequately perceived phonemes" (p. 79).

According to Albert et al., in repetition Wernicke's aphasics "fail miserably"; the errors consist of verbal or phonemic paraphasias or a combination. Written word comprehension impairment parallels the auditory word comprehension difficulty, and oral reading is also said to be similarly disturbed—although there are fragmentary reports of patients where the investigators were impressed by how well preserved oral reading was in comparison to other performances (Hier and Mohr 1977; Heilman, Rothi, Companella, and Wolfson 1979).

Hécaen (1972) argued that two subtypes of Wernicke's aphasia could be distinguished. Some subjects had a primary difficulty in phonemic decoding; as a result auditory comprehension was poor and repetition was disturbed both with real words and nonwords. Written word comprehension (which, Hécaen claims, does not involve phonemic decoding) is much better than auditory comprehension. Other subjects have a central difficulty in verbal semantic comprehension, which causes equal disturbance in comprehension of written and spoken words; repetition of real words is better than repetition of nonwords. Writing to dictation is better for real words than nonwords, but spontaneous writing is "filled with abundant paragraphias."

It seems likely that, as Hécaen emphasizes (following Wernicke and Lichtheim), word comprehension systems could break down for a variety of reasons; results that depend on the average scores of groups of Wernicke's aphasics are unlikely to allow us to distinguish different levels of comprehension impairment. As we saw, the Boston neuropsychologists identify Wernicke's aphasics by the characteristics they show in their spontaneous speech *production*; this approach to diagnosis is unlikely to distinguish between different levels of breakdown in *comprehension*. These will be distinguished more productively in terms of the properties of the systems for comprehension of written and spoken words.

2 Word deafness

Like Wernicke's aphasics, patients with word deafness also have disturbed auditory comprehension. Where the disorder is pure, they differ from Wernicke's aphasics by having good reading comprehension (relative to their auditory comprehension) and unimpaired spontaneous speech (although almost all the recorded cases have some degree of word retrieval deficit; see Goldstein 1974). To distinguish this from a peripheral deafness, Bonvincini (1905) emphasized that nonverbal audiometric testing of hearing should be normal (or nearly so). Word deafness then, is used to describe a selective disorder of auditory comprehension. Some patients, in addition to a difficulty in understanding spoken language, have difficulty in interpreting or identifying nonspeech sounds; these patients are sometimes described as having a general 'auditory agnosia' of which their word deafness is only one element.

The classical German literature employed a distinction, which had been drawn by Ziehl (1896), between word sound deafness (*Wortlauttaubheit*) and word meaning deafness (*Wortsinntaubheit*). In word sound deafness, the difficulty lies in auditory word sound recognition; in Goldstein's (1974) term there is an 'auditory agnosia for speech'. In the early cases, patients demonstrated that they could perceive word sounds, by repeating or writing to dictation single phonemes, while they could not understand, write, or repeat whole words (e.g., Ziehl 1896; Henneberg 1906). More recent case reports mostly concern patients who seem to have no ability to repeat words or isolated speech sounds (e.g., Klein and Harper 1956; Shoumaker, Ajax, and Schenkenberg 1977). Goldstein (1906) had pointed out that a patient might be unable to *repeat* a word or sound, but nevertheless be able to *perceive* it. Fortunately some of the more careful investigators have investigated word sound perception in other ways—for example by same/different judgments on phonemes—and demonstrated that here, too, patients' phoneme perception is impaired (e.g., Auerbach, Allard, Naeser, Alexander, and Albert 1982; Saffran, Marin, and Yeni-Komshian 1976).

In word meaning deafness, the patient can perceive the sound pattern of the word but fails to retrieve its meaning. Evidence of intact word sound perception is usually taken to be that the patient can repeat the word correctly. In some cases the patient is reported to be able to write down the words that s/he cannot understand, and then read that word in order to understand it (e.g., Bramwell 1897; Morton 1980a; Kohn and Friedman 1986). Other patients who have been presented in the literature as cases of pure' word meaning deafness are disturbed in both written and spoken word comprehension (e.g., Symonds 1953; Yamadori and Albert 1973). While it is clearly necessary to have some perceptual representation of a word so as to be able to repeat it, or write it to dictation, it is not necessary to recognize the word lexically to do so: confronted with nonwords, most normal literate adults can repeat them aloud or write them to dictation. One can be sure that a patient has recognized a word in a lexicon of word forms only if the routine used with nonwords would not yield a correct result with that item. Words whose spellings are not unambiguously specified by their sound can only be spelled correctly using word-specific knowledge; this lexical knowledge can only be available after the word is recognized. Thus '/jɒt/' if a nonword would probably be spelled YOT or YOTT; to retrieve the spelling YACHT requires that the word itself has been identified. In three cases of word meaning deafness the patients were able to spell an irregularly spelled word that they could not understand. For one of these patients—Morton's Gail—there is only one example of this (the word PLOUGH). For the other two patients there are two examples: for Kohn and Friedman's HN the words THIGH and KNEE, and for Bramwell's patient the words COME and EDINBURGH. Although between these patients there are very few examples of correctly spelled but uncomprehended words with a *highly* irregular relationship between sound and spelling, relatively few words in English have spellings that are uniquely specified by their pronunciation (see Hatfield and Patterson 1983). Therefore consistently accurate writing to dictation of uncomprehended words will almost certainly indicate that the auditorily presented words have been lexically identified. In these cases, the process of semantic access appears to be interrupted after word recognition has been achieved.

Traditional accounts of word meaning deafness do not distinguish between impairments in auditory lexical representations and post-lexical impairments in semantic access. Kohn and Friedman (1986) try to introduce a distinction of this kind between word meaning deafness of the form described by Morton and by Bramwell (where the lexical word form is correctly accessed), and patients who can repeat words by relying on a nonlexical phonological representation of a heard word but who cannot access the word's representation in an auditory input lexicon. As an example of this second type of disorder, they offer the case of a patient who could repeat but could not spell words that he could not understand; Kohn and Friedman take his failure to spell the words as evidence that he has not accessed the correct word form in the input lexicon. Unfortunately this conclusion is not warranted; the patient could have failed in spelling due to some postlexical disruption in the spelling process. They did not test more directly whether the patient could access lexical representations from heard words, by for example presenting him with an auditory lexical decision task; this would require him to discriminate real, familiar words from phonotactically possible nonwords, which requires, at least, access to stored representations in an input lexicon.

Accounts of word deafness are not easy to evaluate. All of the proposed cases of word meaning deafness rely on accounts of the patients' responses to very small numbers of stimuli; in many, if not all, cases there was some degree of impairment in written word comprehension in addition to the deficit in auditory word comprehension. The reports of cases of word sound deafness are in some ways more satisfactory; the disturbance of auditory comprehension is often total—in relation to speech the patients act as if deaf—while they can easily hear nonspeech sounds. Klein and Harper's (1956) subject described how he could hear everything, "even a leaf falling," but speech "is like a wall between, like a gramophone, boom, boom, jumbled together like foreign folks speaking in the distance. You feel it should be louder but when anyone shouts it is still more confusing" (p. 113). But, as we have shown, even in cases of word sound deafness the testing of phoneme perception has been unsystematic and anecdotal, with the exceptions of the meticulous investigations by Saffran et al. and Auerbach et al. of their patients' difficulties in phoneme perception and discrimination.

It should be evident that while ability to repeat sounds requires some ability to perceive them, failure in repetition need not implicate any defect in word sound perception; word (or nonword) repetition processes may be disturbed in a variety of different ways. Testing of the processes of word perception and recognition cannot afford to make the assumption that postlexical or sublexical repetition and writing processes are necessarily intact. Moreover, word perception could break down at a number of different levels. Word sound identification can be examined by testing patients with minimal pairs, or by examining categorical perception of phonemes. Deciding whether a stimulus is a real word or not requires at least access to phonological representations at a lexical level; this can be tested in auditory lexical decision tasks. Access to central representations of word meaning can be tested with a range of traditional word comprehension tasks. In testing these levels, we have to be aware of the importance of 'top-down' processes. Normal subjects are able to reconstruct clear perceptual representations of speech on the basis of extraordinarily degraded input; clearly central and contextual information can play a role even in the processes of word sound perception (Marslen-Wilson 1984; Warren 1970).

The patient we describe in this book has a specific difficulty in recognition of spoken words. We will argue that word sound perception, as assessed in performance in phoneme minimal pair judgment tasks, is reasonably intact but that he has a specific loss of information in the auditory input lexicon; this results in poor performance in auditory lexical decision and misrecognition of words as phonologically related neighbors. Word repetition and writing to dictation are, however, disturbed in other ways and therefore cannot be used as ways of testing his auditory perceptual abilities. Thus MK represents the first clear case of a certain kind of word deafness caused by a degraded input lexicon, which is neither the classical word sound deafness nor word meaning deafness.

3 Semantic errors in repetition

Many authors have claimed that word deafness is extremely rare, and its supposed existence depends on a small number of anecdotally described patients. The existence of patients who make semantic errors in single word repetition that are unrelated to the target word in sound is even more precarious; this may reflect either the fact that it is a very rare symptom, or that it is rarely reported because it is not thought to be of any particular interest. Only since Marshall and Newcombe (1966, 1973) drew attention to the significance of semantic errors in single word reading (part of the symptomcomplex called 'deep dyslexia'; see Coltheart, Patterson and Marshall, 1980), have modern reports of patients who make the corresponding errors in auditory-verbal repetition emerged. We have managed to find only seven reports of patients of this kind;[1] some of these case reports are very fragmentary. These seven cases and our sources on them are listed in table 1; two of the patients (PS and GL) were first reported as cases of word deafness, and the others as having a disorder of repetition.

This symptomcomplex has been given many different names. Morton (1980b), emphasizing the similarity with 'deep dyslexia,' refers to patients who make semantic errors in word repetition as showing 'the auditory analogue of deep dyslexia'. We have avoided this term for two reasons: (i) it implies a priori that there will be a similarity in theory and practice between these patients and 'deep dyslexics'; we would prefer our account to be motivated by the data from our patient; (ii) oral reading is the production of a spoken response to a written stimulus (a cross-modal task); the most plausible auditory analogue of this is the production of a written response to a spoken stimulus (ie writing to dictation). From this viewpoint the auditory analogue of deep dyslexia is deep dysgraphia; if the term is open to multiple interpretation it is too ambiguous to be useable.

Michel and Andreewsky (1983) suggest 'deep dysphasia'. This too seems inappropriate. The term 'dysphasia' is often taken to imply a problem with all language tasks; the symptom we are concerned with occurs simply in word repetition, which is a task no more (or less) central to language than word reading.

---

1. Some other case reports concern patients who have features in common with the patients described here (e.g., Cruze, cited by Morton 1980b; Nolan and Caramazza 1982; McCarthy and Warrington 1984). None, however, is reported to make phonologically unrelated semantic errors in single word repetition, so they are not included here.

Table 1
Cases of patients who make semantic errors in single word repetition

a. P. S. reported by Goldstein (1906) and described as case 7 in Goldstein (1948)

b. B. F. reported by Goldblum (1979, 1980); this patient's reading is described by Goldblum (1985), and, under the initials F. R. A., by Kremin (1980)

c. M. A. L. reported by Goldblum (1979, 1980)

d. M. R. reported by Michel (1979) and commented on and interpreted by Morton (1980b) and Michel and Andreewsky (1983)

e. G. L. reported by Metz-Lutz and Dahl (1984)

f. M. C. H. reported by Marshall (1982) and Newcombe and Marshall (1984) Elaborated on by Marshall (1987) and Marshall and Newcombe (1988)

g. N. Z. reported by Duhamel and Poncet (1986)

Marshall (1987) introduces a term of uncertain origin—'deep dysrepetonia'. If we are to continue the nineteenth-century custom of giving Greek names to neuropsychological disorders, we would have to use 'deep dyspallilogia'. In Greek, repetition is 'pallilogia' (literally speaking after). We doubt, though, whether this term would catch on, so we prefer to be as neutral and descriptive as possible, by simply describing the symptom-semantic errors in repetition.

Table 2 summarizes the available information on the factors affecting single word repetition in the seven patients reported in the literature as showing semantic errors in repetition. Only in relation to nonword repetition do we have knowledge about all the patients: PS, MR, MCH, and NZ were apparently unable to repeat nonwords correctly, while the other three managed some nonword repetition but were very much worse than with real words. Only three patients were asked to repeat single sounds (which were not real words); neither PS, MR, nor GL could do this. In all five cases where we have information, these patients were worse at repeating abstract words than concrete ones, although with BF and MAL the difference is not marked. In addition BF, MAL, and NZ are reported to be worse at repeating long words than short ones;[2] in contrast MR apparently performs better with longer words, although no systematic study of the effect of word length on his repetition has been published.

In oral word reading, deep dyslexic patients make errors of four major types: semantic (e.g., TABLE → 'chair'), inflectional/derivational errors (e.g., FISHED → 'fishing'), visual (e.g., COD → 'God'), and function word substitu-

2. Duhamel and Poncet (1986) warn that the differences between words of different lengths may reflect effects of word frequency in their lists, which were not controlled. Since it also appears that they did not consider degree of concreteness (other than judging that all the words were concrete), their results should not be given too much weight.

Table 2
Some properties of repetition by patients who make semantic errors in single word repetition

	PS	BF	MAL	MR	GL	MCH	NZ
Repetition of single sounds	Failed	—	—	Failed*	Failed*	—	—
Repetition of nonwords/unfamiliar words	Cannot	17%	32%	Cannot	12%	Failed*	Cannot
Worse at abstract words than concrete words	—	58%v68%	83%v97%	Yes	Yes*	—	40%v89%
Word length effects	—	Short > long	Short > long	Long > short*	—	—	Short > long
Word class effects	—	—	—	Poor with 'function words'	—	—	Function words as bad as abstract words

—No information available
*Personal communication.

tions (e.g., WAS → 'them'). Morton suggests that, by analogy with the deep dyslexics, we would expect the corresponding error types in repetition with patients who make semantic errors. These would consist of semantic errors, inflectional/derivational errors, function word substitutions and, in place of visual errors, real words that are phonologically/auditorily related to the target. One might, in addition, anticipate that articulatory errors might occur in production, resulting in phonologically related nonwords. The available evidence on the occurrence of these error types is assembled in table 3. Where errors of a particular kind have not been reported, we cannot be sure whether they occurred; only where it is claimed, in print, that particular types of errors were absent do we mark them as not occurring. For four patients (PS, MR, GL, and NZ) semantic errors make up the overwhelming majority of the errors the patients made, when they made any kind of response. With other patients there was a greater range of errors. However there is only one report of function word substitutions (NZ), and phonologically related real word errors are only reported to occur with any frequency with BF and MAL; but this may reflect the biases of the case reports and the test stimuli rather than genuinely reflecting the nonoccurrence of particular error types. The five patients where there is most detailed information are all French (BF, MAL, MR, GL, NZ). Testing for impairments in 'function word' processing is particularly difficult in French as the majority of short function words are homophonic with content words; as a result of this limitation, only Michel (1979) and Duhamel and Poncet, 1986) have been able to identify, with any confidence, a difficulty in function word repetition. As a result, we cannot be sure whether a difficulty in function word repetition with function word substitution errors occurs frequently with, or even always with, semantic errors in repetition.

In speech production all these patients are described as fluent, with a wide variety of grammatical constructions and function words; with PS, GL, and MCH the reports mention that there was evidence of word-finding difficulties (circumlocutions, vague terms, abandoned structures, etc.) in their speech. MR produced many phonological errors and neologisms (i.e., nonwords unrelated to any identifiable target). The performance of these patients in related tasks of word comprehension and production are shown in table 4. Auditory comprehension is poor in all cases except MAL, where it is said to be "relatively good." Written word comprehension is nearly always better.

The data on oral word reading are particularly intriguing. Two patients (MCH and BF) can clearly be described as 'surface dyslexic'. They are both better at reading words whose spelling accurately represents their phonology ('regular words', e.g., FEW, KERNEL) than with words where the phonology is not predictable from the spelling ('irregular words', e.g., SEW, COLONEL). Their reading errors appear to reflect reliance on a system which

Table 3

Some types of errors in single word repetition by patients who make semantic errors

Patient PS

Semantic errors
     'Dorf' → 'Haus'   ('village' → 'house')
     'Gott' → 'Kirche'   ('God' → 'church')
     'Maus' → 'Katze'   ('mouse' → 'cat')
     'Flasche' → 'Trichter'   ('bottle' → 'funnel')

Inflectional/derivational errors
     'Tinte' → 'Tintenfass'   ('ink' → 'inkwell')

Phonologically related real word errors
    Do not occur

Phonologically related nonword errors
    Do not occur

Omissions (no response)
    Common

Patient BF

Semantic errors**
     'synagogue' → 'église'   ('synagogue' → 'church')
     'mauvais' → 'mal'   ('bad' → 'pain')
     'saphir' → 'diamant'   ('sapphire' → 'diamond')
     'reptile' → 'serpent'   ('reptile' → 'snake')
     Make up 9% of errors with real words

Inflectional/derivational errors
    Not reported

Phonologically related real word errors
    Frequent: make up 21% of errors with real words

Phonologically related nonword errors
    Frequent: make up 33% of errors with real words

Omissions (no response)
    Make up 12% of errors with real words

Patient MAL

Semantic errors
    Frequent: make up 20% of errors with real words

Inflectional/derivational errors
    Occasional: make up 3% of errors with real words

Phonologically related real word errors
    Infrequent: make up 6% of errors with real words

Phonologically related nonword errors
    Frequent: make up 31% of errors with real words

Omissions (no response)
    Common: make up 32% of errors with real words

Patient MR

Semantic errors
     'coucher' → 'dormir'   ('to lie down' → 'to sleep')
     'noyau' → 'pêche'   ('nut' → 'peach')
     'ballon' → 'cerf-volant' ('balloon' → 'kite')
     'crabe' → 'homard'   ('crab' → 'lobster')

Inflectional/derivational errors
     'mangerais' → 'manger'   ('eat' 1st person singular future → 'eat' infinitive)

Table 3 (continued)

'lu' → 'lire'	('read' past participle → 'read' infinitive)
'jardinier' → 'jardin'	('gardener' → 'garden')

Phonologically related real word errors
  Very rare
Phonologically related nonword errors
  Very common
Omissions (no response)
  Common, especially with abstract words and function words

Patient GL

Semantic errors
  All errors in single word repetition: no other types of error occur (but only tested with 50 items; no examples given)
Inflectional/derivational errors
  Not reported
Phonologically related errors
  Occur only with nonword stimuli
Omissions (no response)
  Rare

Patient MCH

Semantic errors
  'book' → 'from reading'
  'nephew' → 'father ... mother'
  'college' → 'oh yes ... to learn'
  'metronome' → 'automatic'
Inflectional/derivational errors
  Do not occur*
Phonologically related errors
  'cow' → 'cry ... crew'
  'port' → 'pork'
  'nut' → 'to nuck'
Omissions (no response)
  Not reported

Patient NZ

No examples of NZ's errors were reported
Semantic errors
  Frequent: make up 43% of errors with content words
Inflectional/derivational errors
  Occasional: make up 9% of errors with content words
Phonologically related errors
  Frequent: make up 25% of errors with content words
Function word substitutions
  Frequent: make up 73% of errors with function words
Omissions (no response)
  Occur only with abstract words and function words

* Personal communication
** Goldblum presents BF's and MAL's semantic errors together; thus, some or all of these examples of semantic errors may in fact have been made by MAL.

Table 4
Other features of language performance by patients who make semantic errors in single word repetition

	PS	BF	MAL	MR	GL	MCH	NZ
Auditory word comprehension	Poor	Poor	'relatively good'	Poor	Very poor	'Severely impaired'	'Relatively preserved'
Auditory lexical decision	Poor	—	—	Very poor*	Good	—	Poor
Written word comprehension	Good "in general"	Relatively good	—	Unimpaired (with concrete words)	Good	Impaired (esp. with homophones)	'Excellent'
Oral word reading	Good	Surface dyslexic	—	Very slow. Phonemically inaccurate	Good	Surface dyslexic	—
Writing to dictation	Can write if he can repeat	"elements of both surface and deep dysgraphia"	'total agraphia'	Semantic errors	Very poor. Semantic errors*	Deep dysgraphic	—
Oral picture naming	Poor: errors are omissions	Good	—	Very poor. Non-word responses	Good. No semantic errors*	Poor: errors are semantic	Disturbed: errors are semantic or phonol. related nonwords
Written picture naming	—	—	—	Good	Good. No semantic errors*	—	'Perfect'
Digit span	—	4 digits	—	1 digit	—	—	Pointing span is 2

—No evidence available
*Personal communication

uses knowledge of the relationship between orthography and phonology; these errors are therefore 'phonologically plausible' renderings of the written letter string (e.g., reading SEW as 'sue' or COLONEL as '/'kɒlənəl/'). The other three patients are reported to read aloud relatively well; but unless they were specifically given irregularly spelled words to read, the features of surface dyslexia would probably not have been noticed. In two cases (MR and GL) the investigators could find no evidence of surface dyslexic errors (Michel, Metz-Lutz, personal communication). The problem of identifying surface dyslexia would be particularly acute with the German patient PS, because irregular words in German are almost all foreign loan words, and are relatively infrequent (Scheerer 1987). These data provoke a question: Is there some kind of functional association between semantic errors in repetition and surface dyslexia? And, if there is, is there an underlying information processing deficit common to both tasks? MK, the patient we describe in this book is, like both BF and MCH, surface dyslexic. In the light of his pattern of performance we will argue in the final section, that there is a specific central semantic deficit that causes him both to make semantic errors in repetition and to be surface dyslexic in oral word reading.

In writing to dictation, several patients are said to be 'deep dysgraphic'— among other features, they make semantic errors and are unable to write nonwords. Or, as Goldstein claims for his patient PS, the properties of writing are the same as the properties of repetition; this amounts to the same claim in a different form. Like these patients, our subject was a deep dysgraphic; we will argue again in the last section that the association is no accident. Common impairments underlie the disorders in oral repetition and writing to dictation.

Finally table 4 demonstrates that there is no necessary association between the occurrence of semantic errors in repetition and difficulties in word retrieval in spoken and written picture naming; in some cases the naming deficit is severe while for others there is only a mild degree of impairment. The data on digit span is striking: patient BF who is impaired in repeating nonwords or abstract words is nevertheless able to repeat strings of four digits. A span of four digits is clearly defective relative to normal people, but a restricted span cannot be a sufficient explanation of semantic errors in repetition; this is because the patients for whom a restricted repetition span is the prominent problem, the patients with disorders of short term memory, do not make semantic errors in immediate repetition of single words (see Shallice, 1979b; Shallice and Vallar, 1989 for reviews). There is, therefore, a double dissociation between restricted repetition span and semantic errors in repetition. In another paper we have analyzed MK's short term memory abilities (Howard and Franklin 1989); we argue that, although his repetition span is one item at best, he has a prelexical phonological input store of approximately normal capacity.

Duhamel and Poncet (1986) show that their patient NZ performs poorly in phoneme discrimination and identification. Like Goldstein (1906) before them, they suggest that a difficulty in phoneme perception might underlie the semantic errors in repetition. It is not clear how this might happen; phoneme misperception is a natural explanation of phonologically related errors in repetition; but without some additional mechanisms it cannot account for semantic errors. Furthermore the patients with word sound deafness (who all misperceive phonemes) make phonological, but not semantic, errors in repetition (see, e.g., Saffran et al. 1976; Auerbach et al. 1982). And, as we shall show in our report with MK, semantic errors in repetition can occur with patients who show no significant impairment in discriminating phonemes.

We have reviewed the patterns of impairment in all the patients who make semantic errors in single word repetition for two reasons. First, we wanted to assemble information that is in many different forms and in which the authors may have focused originally on some other aspect of the patients' disorders. Second, we wanted to establish whether any other features necessarily or commonly co-occurred with the semantic errors. Conclusions from the available case reports must inevitably be tentative, but there are a number of features that appear always to accompany semantic errors in repetition: poor nonword repetition; some kind of disorder in writing to dictation; and, in some patients, a deficit in oral word reading. Unfortunately all the case reports are incomplete in vital respects so we cannot be sure about many of the relevant details.

Despite this we can come to two conclusions about the repetition routines available to these patients. First, they cannot use a repetition routine that operates on unfamiliar words (they can't repeat nonwords). They must therefore be using a lexical routine in repetition. Second, the lexical routine that they use involves semantic mediation, on at least some occasions. There are two sources of evidence for this: (i) The occurrence of semantic errors indicates that at some point the information must have been semantically coded. (ii) For some, and possibly all, of the patients success in word repetition is affected by whether a word is abstract or concrete—a semantic factor. We must conclude that these patients are using a semantically mediated lexical routine for word repetition.

There is a group of patients who have defective word repetition and show some features in common with the patients who make semantic errors. These are described by Shallice and Warrington (1977) as 'reproduction conduction aphasics'. A number of recent case histories give quite detailed information about these subjects (McCarthy and Warrington 1984; Caramazza, Miceli, and Villa 1986; Caplan, Vanier, and Baker 1986). All of them are better at repeating real words than nonwords, but none make semantic errors. In word and nonword repetition, errors are phonologically related to the targets. The patients described by McCarthy and Warrington and Caplan et al. seem to have a general phonological output impairment; they are worse at producing long words than short ones, and the same pattern of errors is found in spoken naming and reading aloud as well as repetition. The difficulty with nonwords may simply be because nonword production (which is not supported by a lexical representation) is more vulnerable to an impairment in phonological output. The Caramazza et al. patient IGR made no errors in repeating real words, and even with non-words the impairments was not severe—he repeated 90% of nonwords with four to five phonemes (which seems unlikely to be much worse than normal subjects!). To the extent that there is impairment, Caramazza et al. suggest that there is a difficulty in assembly of nonwords for output; a similar pattern of breakdown is also evident in reading.

Aside from the lack of semantic errors, there are two obvious ways in which these patients differ from those that make semantic errors in repetition. In the 'reproduction conduction aphasics' the natural explanation of the deficit in nonword repetition is at an output level. Several of the patients who make semantic errors in repetition have no difficulty in nonword production in reading (BF, GL, MCH); so a general nonword output problem cannot account for the difficulty in repetition. Second, the impairment with nonword repetition is milder with the reproduction conduction aphasics than the patients who make semantic errors in repetition, four of whom are unable to repeat any nonwords at all. For the latter patients the difficulty with nonwords is not plausibly due to a difficulty with output to which nonwords are more vulnerable. A third difference supports this view: whereas the McCarthy and Warrington and Caplan et al. patients are worse at repeating long words than short ones, Michel's patient MR and our subject MK show the reverse effect. Despite the inadequacies of most of the case reports of patients who make semantic errors in repetition, it is clear that the underlying impairments are rather different from the patients who show the pattern characteristic of reproduction conduction aphasia.

4 *Deep dysgraphia*

Just as patients who make semantic errors in single word repetition appear to rely on a lexical semantic routine in word repetition, patients who make semantic errors in writing to dictation—the 'deep dysgraphics'—appear to rely on a lexical-semantic routine. There are now a variety of reports of patients of this kind (e.g., Newcombe and Marshall 1980 (patient GR); Bub and Kertesz 1982 (JC); Hatfield 1982, 1983, 1985 (PW, DE, BB); Hatfield and Patterson 1984 (DE, BB); Nolan and Caramazza 1982 (BL), 1983 (VS); Byng et al. 1984 (B)). The accounts agree that, in addition to semantic errors, the patients show the following features in writing to dictation:

1. Better at writing concrete words than abstract words.
2. Poor at writing 'function words' as compared to content words.
3. Either very poor or completely abolished performance in writing nonsense words to dictation.
4. May make 'inflectional/derivational errors', 'function word substitutions', and errors that appear to reflect partial lexical knowledge without retrieval of the complete spelling (e.g., 'science' → SCIECE, SCEINE, SCEICE; from Bub and Kertesz 1982, p. 163).

While there is in the available case reports remarkable agreement about the symptoms that these patients can show, there is a variable picture of associated disabilities. Some of these subjects (e.g., GR, PW, BB, DE, VS) are both deep dysgraphic and deep dyslexic, but have no real impairment in single word repetition. One patient, BL, is deep dyslexic and deep dysgraphic, and has some degree of impairment in single item repetition, which is particularly evident with nonwords, although he does not make phonologically unrelated semantic repetition errors. In contrast, Bub and Kertesz's patient JC has no problem in either oral reading or repetition of single words and nonwords. Some of the patients described in the previous section (e.g., BF and MCH) are deep dysgraphic, make semantic errors in repetition, and yet are surface dyslexic! Only one association seems to hold: all patients who make semantic errors in repetition are probably deep dysgraphic, although it is evident from the Bub and Kertesz case of JC that the reverse—that deep dysgraphia implies semantic errors in repetition—is not true. As we shall discuss in part III, this may be a prediction from some versions of lexical theory.

5 Surface dyslexia

As with all the terms we have discussed, different researchers have used their technical terms in subtly different ways. We have suggested elsewhere that surface dyslexia should be used to describe any patient who shows the following two features in oral word reading:

(i) Superior accuracy in reading words with a regular relationship between their orthography and their phonology (e.g., FEW, KERNEL) than matched irregular words whose phonology cannot be deduced from their orthography (SEW, COLONEL).
(ii) A substantial proportion of the misreadings should be phonologically plausible renderings of the written letter string, in terms of the possible relationships between orthography and phonology in the

language (e.g., reading SEW as 'sue' or COLONEL as '/'kɒlənəl/'; Howard and Franklin, 1987).

This description differs radically from Marshall (1976) and Coltheart, Masterson, Byng, Prior, and Riddoch (1983) who have proposed a syndrome of 'surface dyslexia' that can be defined in terms of a variety of features relating not only to oral word reading but also to written word comprehension and writing to dictation. We do not wish to claim that surface dyslexia is a syndrome in the sense that if a patient shows *one* of these symptoms then all the others will invariably be found as well. Instead we would argue, as did many of the individual authors in a book devoted to surface dyslexia (Patterson, Marshall, and Coltheart 1985), that there will be a wide variety of possible patterns of impairment associated with the two symptoms of a regularity effect and phonologically plausible errors in reading.

Taken together, these two symptoms suggest that the patients cannot always use lexically specific information in word reading; where lexical information is missing or unavailable, they have to rely instead on a sublexical reading routine (SLRR) for generating pronunciations for written words. Exactly how such a routine might operate is a matter of debate; two classes of theory have been proposed. Either words are pronounced using a system of rules that express a relationship between orthography and phonology (Coltheart 1978; Patterson and Morton 1985) or the system might generate a pronunciation by analogy with other, similar real words (Glushko 1979; Marcel 1980; Kay and Marcel 1981). In practice these theories may not be very different from each other (Humphreys and Evett 1985; Patterson and Coltheart 1987); our present description of MK does not require us to enter this debate. Descriptions of different surface dyslexic patients make it clear that they may use very different sizes of orthographic segment to generate phonology (see Shallice, Warrington, and McCarthy 1983; Kay and Lesser 1985; Newcombe and Marshall 1985).

However, the claim that surface dyslexics are sometimes forced to rely on a sublexical routine in oral word reading entails the corollary that the lexical routines for deriving word-specific pronunciations from orthography are defective; deficits in lexical reading procedures might occur at one of several different levels (Coltheart and Funnell 1987, distinguish, on theoretical grounds, seven possible loci!). In most of the early reports the difficulty seems to lie at the level of the visual input lexicon; in general these patients are forced to rely on a phonological code generated by the SLRR for semantic access. As a result words are understood as they are (mis)pronounced; the first surface dyslexic patient, JC, described by Marshall and Newcombe (1973), read the word LISTEN as 'Liston ... that's the boxer'. Irregular words, where the SLRR generates the incorrect phonology, are generally misunderstood; where the misreading is a real word, patients will misdefine it as that word (e.g., BEAR → 'something you drink' [i.e., beer]) or, when the misreading is a non-word, the patient will volunteer no meaning (e.g., YACHT → 'that's not a word—/jætʃt/'). In lexical decision tasks with written words the analogous problem is found; irregular words (whose SLRR-generated phonologies usually sound like nonwords) tend to get rejected, while the patients accept many pseudo-homophones (non-words that, when pronounced, sound like real words—e.g., SCURT, KWENE) (Kay and Patterson 1985). Words with homophones will also present a problem: if their meaning is accessed on the basis of a phonological code alone, the patient will be unable to distinguish between meanings that have orthographically distinct spellings. So the patient JC glossed the word BEE as 'to be or not to be, that is the question' (Newcombe and Marshall 1981).

A number of different case studies in Patterson, Marshall, and Coltheart (1985) document individual instances where a patient, while having accessed the incorrect phonology for a word, was nevertheless able to understand the word correctly (see e.g., Deloche, Andreewsky, and Desi 1982; Kay and Patterson 1985; Goldblum 1985; Kremin 1985). For instance, EST (described by Kay and Patterson 1985), defined GAUGE as 'that is something about a railway ... that's as much as I've got, train ... /gɔdʒ/'; for this item EST, despite retrieving the *phonology* for a different word (gorge), provides an appropriate (if partial) *definition* of the correct word (gauge). None of the subjects described was able to consistently provide correct definitions for words that were mispronounced; with the majority of words access to meaning depended on prior phonological recoding. Several authors have suggested that the instances of correct definition and mispronunciation can be attributed to a defect in the lexical reading system at the level of an output phonological lexicon (e.g., Kay and Patterson 1985).

The literature therefore distinguishes two levels of breakdown in a lexical reading process that can underlie surface dyslexia. With an input deficit, both written word comprehension and lexical decision have to rely on phonological recoding. Where there is a deficit in a lexicon of stored phonological word forms (or in access to it), comprehension and lexical decision can be normal irrespective of the way the patient reads the word aloud; we know of no published report of a patient who consistently shows this pattern of impairment.

The patient we will describe in this book has a third, and qualitatively different, kind of impairment to his lexical reading procedure, while his sublexical reading routine is relatively undisturbed. We will demonstrate that MK has a normal visual input lexicon, as demonstrated by normal lexical decision, even for irregular words and pseudo-homophones. MK has a deficit in word comprehension that is especially marked for abstract words; this problem is central, at least in the sense that the same deficit is found in comprehension of both spoken and written words. If his lexical reading routine is specifically semantic (that is he cannot use a lexical but nonsemantic 'direct' route from an orthographic input lexicon to output phonology), he should be particularly inaccurate in reading abstract irregular words. We will show that for MK this is the case; in word reading there is a regularity effect with abstract words but not with concrete words. On these grounds we will argue that his lexical reading routines are defective in at least two ways: first the 'direct route' is unavailable, and second, the point of breakdown in the 'lexical semantic reading routine' is neither at input nor at output, but central.

A simple lexical model for single word processing

Figure 1 illustrates our adaptation of Patterson's (1986) model of lexical organization. It is intended as a partial specification of a theory that will

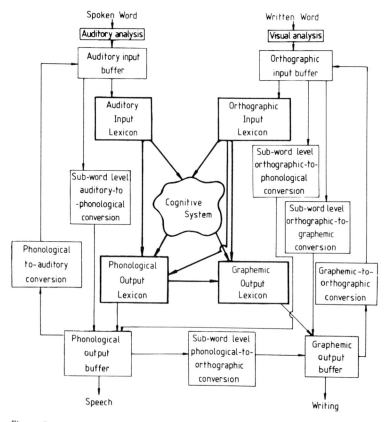

Figure 1
A simple model of single word lexical processing; adapted from Howard and Franklin (1987).

account for performance in a variety of different tasks—repetition, oral reading, writing to dictation, and so on—with single words and nonwords. We do not propose to justify this model here (for discussion and justification of this and related approaches to modeling the organization of lexical and nonlexical processing see Morton 1979 and Monsell 1987a).

The core of the model is comprized of the five central elements—the auditory and orthographic input lexicons, the 'cognitive system', and the phonological and graphemic output lexicons. These five elements all specify lexical (i.e., word-specific), information. In figure 1 all lexical processes and addressing are given bold outlines and arrows. The auditory input lexicon is used to recognize familiar (that is lexically represented) spoken words; the orthographic input lexicon is a recognition device for written words. The phonological output lexicon is the source of a specification of the word's spoken form. The graphemic output lexicon specifies its written form. Representations in the cognitive system specify word meanings as well as knowledge about the concepts involved. At this level there will be specifications of linguistic sentence-level knowledge, but this is not our concern in the present work (see Morton and Patterson 1980).

In addition to lexical transcoding processes there are six different systems that allow conversion between different input and output codes; because these processes do not rely on word-specific whole word information they are able to account for the normal person's ability to perform processing tasks with nonwords. One can, for example, repeat, write to dictation, read aloud or copy nonwords with reasonable accuracy. In figure 1 we have added one process of 'orthographic to graphemic conversion', which was not included in previous versions of this model. The addition accounts for the ability to copy written nonwords presented in a familiar script. (Copying words in an unfamiliar script presumably depends on stroke-by-stroke reproduction involving no processes of letter recognition or production.)

Consider the four tasks of spoken word repetition, writing to dictation, oral word reading, and delayed copying (the written analogue of oral repetition). They all take a word (or nonword) as input and produce the same word as output. For each of them the model provides three possible routines. A sublexical routine converts between the input and output codes and does not depend on whole word lexical knowledge; this system will have to be used with nonwords, but can also be used with real words. Where the conversion between the input and output codes is not a simple 1 : 1 correspondence, relying on a sublexical routine with real words will lead to errors; as for instance in oral word reading in French or English. Then the system allows two different kinds of lexical routine for each of the four tasks: in the 'lexical semantic routines' a word recognized by the input lexicon retrieves information in the cognitive system, which is then used to address the output lexicon. In this routine central semantic representations mediate between input and output. Each task also has a 'direct' (i.e., non-semantic) lexical processing routine. In these routines, words recognized by the input lexicon can be used to address the output lexicon, without accessing central representations in the cognitive system. In the diagram there are direct connections for three of the four tasks: the exception is writing words to dictation where this version of the model requires the phonological output lexicon to be used as an intermediate stage (Patterson 1986, considers the arguments for and against this particular arrangement).

We are concerned with two other kinds of tasks in this book: word comprehension (i.e., access to central semantic representations from a heard or spoken word) and word production (retrieval of a word from an output lexicon, on the basis of a central semantic representation). In principle, both of these tasks are straightforward in relation to this model: there is only one simple routine possible for each task. Unfortunately, real data does not necessarily turn out to be so simple. We will argue that MK's spoken word production is sometimes influenced by a much more complex routine involving (covert) retrieval of the orthographic word form as a stage in its production.

This model is not the only plausible model of lexical processing currently available. In part II we will consider the implications that the data from MK have for some other kinds of lexical theory. For our purposes most of the competing theories suffer from a major practical disadvantage; they tend to be restricted to one domain of processing, such as auditory word recognition or reading words aloud. Morton and Patterson's model has the advantage that it has components to deal with all the tasks with which we are concerned. Within this conceptual framework we now turn to the data from MK's performance in single word processing tasks.

I

MK: An Analysis of Single Word Processing

Chapter 2
Case Description

Medical history

Until he suffered a stroke in September 1982 shortly before his sixty-fifth birthday, MK worked in the oil industry, employed initially by an oil company and more recently working as an independent consultant. He had worked in many different countries.

For many years, MK had suffered from severe left-frontal headaches that had started when he was working in Shanghai in 1949 (The takeover by Mao Dzedong's government in 1949 cannot have been an easy period for an employee of a western oil company in Shanghai.) He also had a long-standing history of hypertension and dizzy spells, as well as gout.

He had two 'fits', in June and September 1982. Nine days after the second of these he had a third fit, after which he fell asleep; when his wife woke him, his speech was incomprehensible. He was admitted to hospital the following day (19 September 1982). On examination he was found to be fully conscious, but with a total receptive aphasia' with jargon output, flushed face, and telangectasia (red patches on the skin). The only motor signs were brisk reflexes in both legs. The following day he became restless and aggressive, and later in the day he had to be taken into intensive care with supraventricular tachycardia, following a probable anterior myocardial infarct.

A CT scan on 24 September 1982 showed that there was an infarct in the left posterior parietal region. In addition there was some degree of generalized cerebral atrophy with enlarged ventricles and several small infarcts.

His progress was uneventful, and MK was discharged on 13 October; his only neurological sign at this point was a severe Wernicke's aphasia, with marked difficulty in auditory comprehension, with fluent and sometimes neologistic speech. He regularly attended speech therapy over the following year and made some improvement. The investigations reported here were performed over the period January 1984 to September 1986.

MK has now retired and lives at home. He has an active social life, and he goes to exhibitions in pursuit of his interest in art; he watches cricket

Patient's Name __M.K.__   Date of rating __29 May 1984__

                                      Rated by __S F.__

APHASIA SEVERITY RATING SCALE

0. No usable speech or auditory comprehension.

1. All communication is through fragmentary expression; great need for inference, questioning and guessing by the listener. The range of information which can be exchanged is limited, and the listener carries the burden of communication.

2. Conversation about familiar subjects is possible with help from the listener. There are frequent failures to convey the idea, but patient shares the burden of communication with the examiner.

3. The patient can discuss <u>almost all everyday problems</u> with little or no assistance. However, reduction of speech and/or comprehension make conversation about certain material difficult or impossible.

4. Some obvious loss of fluency in speech or facility of comprehension, without significant limitation on ideas expressed or form of expression.

5. Minimal discernible speech handicaps; patient may have subjective difficulties which are not apparent to listener.

RATING SCALE PROFILE OF SPEECH CHARACTERISTICS

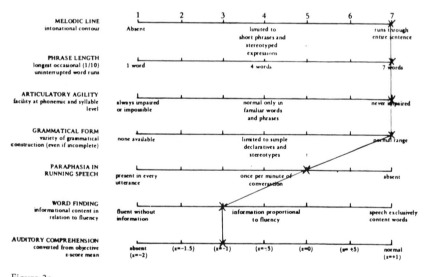

Figure 2a

MK's performance on the Boston Diagnostic Aphasia Examination.

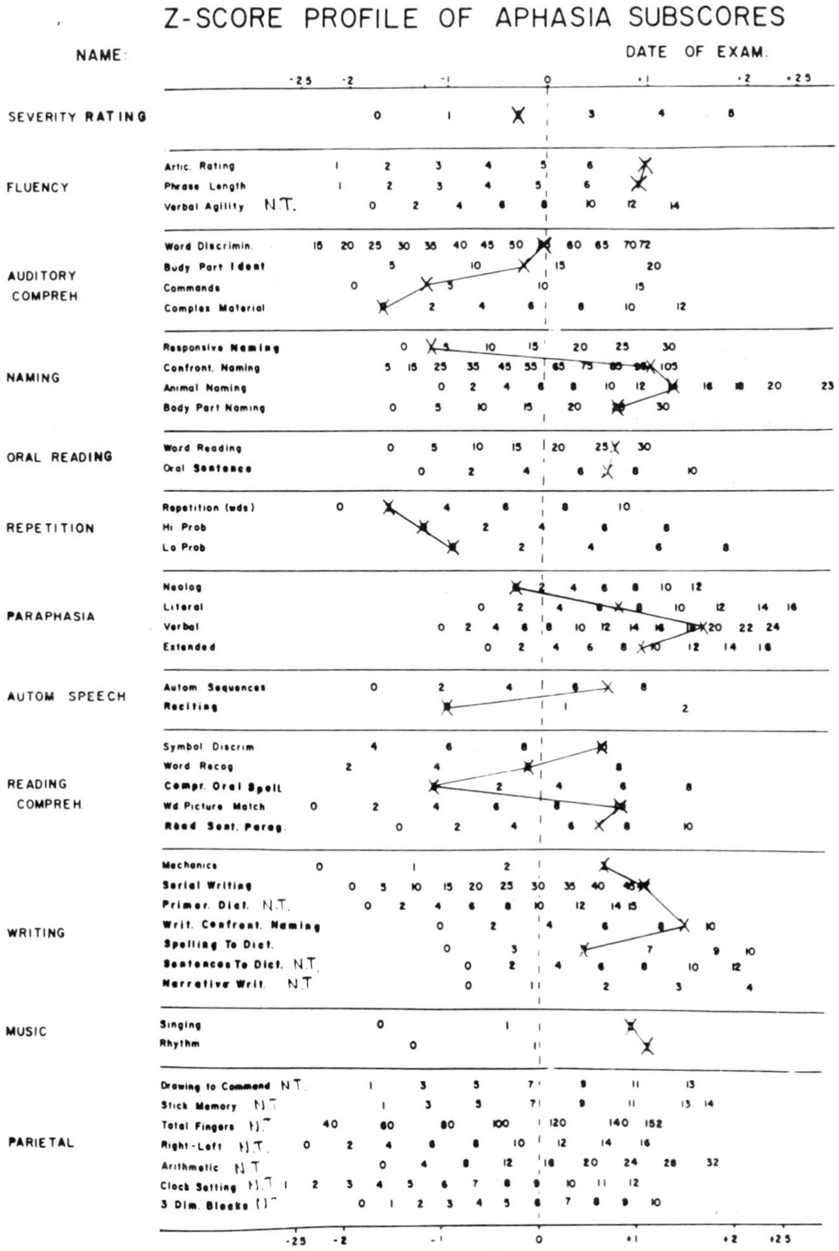

Z-SCORE PROFILE OF APHASIA SUBSCORES

Figure 2b
MK's performance on the Boston Diagnostic Aphasia Examination.

regularly. He still attends a variety of official functions, although he generally avoids situations in which he will be called upon to speak. Despite his language disability, which as we will demonstrate is severe, MK manages to lead a varied and generally active life.

Aphasia Examination

MK was assessed on the Boston Diagnostic Aphasia Examination (Goodglass and Kaplan 1972) on 29 May 1984. The results are summarized in figure 2.

1. *Spontaneous speech* His speech is fluent and employs a wide variety of grammatical constructions; inflections and 'function words' are abundant; paragrammatisms are, however, frequent. Articulation is good; some phonologically related errors occur. Word retrieval problems for both nouns and verbs are evident, with circumlocutions. Describing the BDAE 'cookie theft' picture, MK said,

> So these . . . these like children, young people. They start up with their washing and with their, with their plate. And they want their, they want their jars and cookies. There's her woman; she is mummy. She tries for the family. She is talking with a /'trɒvɪd . . . 'trɪfəd/ and with a dresser. Well they talk themselves. They are with the dresser. They they, there is the sink s-ɪ-ɴ-/ki/, with water. And there is a window with a wind [i.e. /wɪnd/]. She is cleaning the /'krækərɪ/, crockery. But has troublesome, troublesome.

2. *Auditory comprehension* is severely disturbed. The BDAE scores suggest that single word comprehension is somewhat better preserved than understanding of longer material. With single words, MK made no errors with objects, actions and shapes, and performed worse with letters (2/6), colors (3/6), and numbers (4/6).

3. *Naming* is reasonably good, except for naming to spoken description ('responsive naming'), where MK had difficulty in understanding the descriptions.

4. *Repetition* was severely impaired even with single words. With phrases he managed none correctly; there were semantic errors (e.g, 'You should not tell her' → 'I mustn't talk'), and auditorily related errors (e.g., 'Pry the tin lid off' → 'private telephone').

5. *Reading* aloud was reasonably accurate, and written word comprehension was good, although MK was unable to understand words spelled aloud to him. *Writing* was fluent, and relatively good.

Conclusion

MK shows a pattern of impairment in his spontaneous speech which is, according to Goodglass and Kaplan (1972), characteristic of a Wernicke's aphasic. The test scores indicate a severe deficit in auditory comprehension and repetition and all other tasks that involve spoken input, while naming, oral reading, and writing are only mildly impaired.

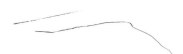

Chapter 3
Oral Reading of Single Words

The model of lexical processing distinguishes three possible routines that could be used for reading words aloud (see figure 3). There is a 'sublexical reading routine' (SLRR), which takes letter strings and, parsing them into sub-word units, finds the corresponding phonology (the process of 'sub-word level orthographic-to-phonological conversion'), which is assembled into a phoneme sequence and articulated. This routine generates, in Patterson's (1981) terminology, 'assembled phonology'. A system of this kind will allow skilled readers to read unfamiliar words—nonwords, or those real words that a reader has never been exposed to before. It can also be used to read real words, and where their orthography corresponds to their phonology, it will yield the correct pronunciation.

To deal with words having an exceptional correspondence between spelling and phonology, the skilled reader will need a system that can capture the lexically specific quirks of English spelling; that can specify that YACHT is pronounced /jɒt/ and SEW /səʊ/. That is, there must be an 'addressed' phonology.

The lexical model provides two different ways of addressing word-specific phonological specifications. There is a 'direct route' where familiar words are recognized as whole units in an orthographic input lexicon; this, in turn, addresses the corresponding entries in the phonological output lexicon, which specify the word's pronunciation. This routine does not require accessing a word's meaning at an intermediate stage.

In contrast, the second lexical route to phonology involves accessing a central representation corresponding to the word, on the basis of word recognition in the orthographic input lexicon. This central representation, which specifies a word's meaning, addresses an entry in the phonological output lexicon.

Whether there is compelling evidence for two distinct routes to addressed phonology is a matter of dispute. Funnell (1983a) and Coltheart (1985), for example, assert that a 'direct route' must exist, while Howard (1985a) argues that the evidence is far from compelling. For our discussion we will assume that either routine can exist. Either of them will yield the correct pronounciations for any real word, whatever its spelling-to-sound relation-

Table 5
Nonword reading: the effects of word length (60 nonwords presented twice)

	Nonword phoneme length		
	3	4	5–6
	n = 9	n = 31	n = 20
Proportion correct	0.94	0.87	0.70

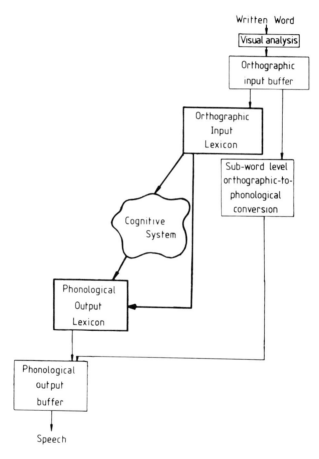

Figure 3
Three routines for oral word reading; all other components of the model are omitted.

ship, but will not be able to cope with unfamiliar words. However, only the 'semantic reading routine' should be sensitive to semantically related variables (such as a word's concreteness, or its part of speech), while the direct route should only be affected by nonsemantic but word-specific variables such as word frequency. Bub, Cancelliere, and Kertesz (1985) have argued that a defective 'direct reading routine' is more likely to yield correct pronunciation for high frequency words than for low frequency words; their patient—who they claim was reading via a direct route—was more accurate with high frequency than low frequency irregular words.

Reading nonwords aloud

MK was asked to read a set of 30 nonwords (taken from Coltheart 1980a); half were pseudo-homophones (e.g., FUE, WUN) and half were not (e.g., FOO, MUN). He read 25/30 correctly; three errors were on pseudo-homophones (e.g., BIE → '/bi/'), and two errors on non-pseudo-homophones (FOO → '/gu/'). This is good performance and suggests that the sublexical reading routine (SLRR) is reasonably intact, at least with single syllable nonwords.

To examine MK's nonword reading slightly more closely, we presented him with a set of sixty nonwords of one or two syllables, which varied in length from three to six phonemes. These were presented on two occasions mixed with real words. Overall, .82 of responses were correct (table 5); there was no effect of syllable length, but there was a significant effect of phoneme length (Jonckheere trend test, $z = 2.42$, $p < .01$). So while MK is reasonably accurate in reading short nonwords, his accuracy declines with longer words. These results are compatible with the view that MK has a 2–3% probability of misreading any individual phoneme in a nonword; with increasing numbers of phonemes in the (non)word, the probability that all will be correct declines. It is clear that, while MK manages reasonable accuracy in nonword reading, his performance is not perfect. But, like MK, normal subjects do not read nonwords perfectly—Glushko (1979, experiment 1), for instance, found a mean error rate of 14% for normal subjects reading single syllable items, in lists of mixed words and nonwords.[3]

Reading irregularly spelled words

If MK were reading real words by a SLRR, he would (i) be worse at reading 'irregular' words than matched regular words, and (ii) make phonologically

3. Although Glushko does not report the nature of the errors, we suspect that they may have been of different kinds. Normal subjects reading nonwords rarely make 'letter substitution' errors of the kind FOO → '/gu/'; more typically their errors involve vowels that can have different realizations depending on their orthographic context (Masterson 1985).

Table 6
The effects of regularity on oral word reading

(i) Words from Coltheart et al. (1979)

	N	Proportion correct	Examples
Regular words	39	.90	SHRUG, PINE
Irregular words	39	.67	SHOVE, PINT

(Fisher exact test, z = 2.17, p < .02)

(ii) Words from Parkin (1982)

	N	Proportion correct	Examples
Regular words	33	.91	DRUG, ORGAN
'Minor correspondences'	33	.82	AUNT, STEAK
Very irregular words	33	.52	CAFE, LEVER

(Jonckheere trend test, z = 3.52, p < .001)

(iii) Words from Glushko (1979)

(eliminating 4 words that are regular in Southern British Standard pronunciation; lists presented twice)

	N	Proportion correct	Examples
Regular consistent words	156	.94	BOND, DEAL
Regular inconsistent words	78	.88	MOTH, LEAF
Irregular inconsistent words	78	.73	BOTH, DEAF

(Chi square (2) = 21.36, p < .001)

(iv) Words from Bauer and Stanovich (1980)

	N	Proportion correct	Examples
Regular words	100	.85	CLICK, FANCY
Irregular words	100	.72	BLOOD, HONEST

(Fisher exact test, z = 2.06, p < .02)

Table 7
Errors in oral reading of the regular and irregular words (from Colheart et al., 1979)

	Irregular words	Regular words
Phonologically plausible errors	AUNT → '/ɔnt/'	SPEAR → '/spɛɑ/'
	GONE → '/gəʊn/'	
	MORTGAGE → '/'mɔtgeɪdʒ/'	
	SEW → '/su/'	
	LOSE → '/ləʊz/'	
	PROVE → '/prəʊv ... prʌv/'	
	MOVE → '/məʊv/'	
Other errors	SUBTLE → 'sublet'	TEETH → 'tooth'
	BUILD → '/hɪld/'	PROTEIN → '/'pruteɪn/'
	ANSWER → '/'ɔnsə/'	CAPSULE → '/'kɒpsjul/'
	SCARCE → '/spɑs ... slɑs/'	
	THOROUGH → '/'θəʊmɒn/'	
	CIRCUIT → '/'sɜkʌt/'	

Table 8
The effects of word imageability on oral word reading

(i) **Words from Coltheart (1980a)**

	N	Proportion correct	Examples
High imageability words	28	.89	HAND, OFFICE
Low imageability words	28	.71	FACT, MOMENT

(ii) **List of high and low imageability words of high and low frequency from Howard (1987)**

	N	Proportion correct	Examples
Low imageability, high frequency words	20	.85	IDEA, ANSWER
Low imageability, low frequency words	20	.85	SPAN, PARDON
High imageability, high frequency words	20	1.00	ROAD, DOCTOR
High imageability, low frequency words	20	.95	HAWK, INFANT

(iii) **List of high and low imageability words matched exactly for word frequency and letter length**

	N	Proportion correct	Examples
High imageability words	100	.94	SKIRT, GRASS, BOMB
Low imageability words	100	.91	BLAME, FAULT, SOUL

plausible reading errors (e.g., BEAR → 'beer', or MORTGAGE → '/mɔtgeɪʤ/').
He was therefore given four published lists of matched regular and irregular words for oral word reading.

The results are shown in table 6. With all four lists, reading of regular words is significantly better than reading of irregular words. The errors from one of these lists are shown in table 7. It is clear that a substantial proportion of his errors are phonologically plausible renderings of the letter string.

MK must, therefore, must be using a SLRR for reading real words on at least some occasions. However, it is also clear that lexical reading processes are by no means entirely abolished, since with all lists he reads a substantial proportion of irregular words correctly. On these occasions at least, the word's phonology must have been lexically retrieved.

The effects of word imageability on oral word reading

Since MK sometimes reads using a lexical routine, MK was asked to read matched sets of high and low imageability words.

The results on three matched lists are presented in table 8; the matching data for the last two lists are given in appendix 1. On the lists from

Coltheart (1980a) and Howard (1987) there are effects of imageability that approach significance (list 1, Fisher exact test, $z = 1.33$, $p = .09$; list 2, $z = 1.57$, $p = .06$). Unfortunately, although matched for frequency and letter length these lists are not matched for spelling regularity, which is obviously crucial in this case; both lists have more irregular words in the low imageability lists, thus confounding the effects of regularity and imageability.

MK was therefore presented with a third list of 100 'low imageability' words and 100 'high imageability' words matched exactly for word frequency and word letter length, where there were approximately equal proportions of regular and irregular words in each list. The results (table 8) show that once word regularity is controlled, word imageability does not affect performance (Fisher exact, $z = 0.54$, $p = .29$).

Part of speech effects in reading

MK was asked to read three different lists of content and function words; matching data for the last two lists are given in appendix 1. The list used by Patterson (1979) is of 60 content words and 60 function words approximately matched in word frequency and exactly matched in word letter length. The second list is compiled from the imageability range where content and function words overlap (i.e., in the MRC psycholinguistic database (Coltheart 1981) in the range 270–350). It consists of all words from that range of imageability values that (i) can be unambiguously categorized as 'content' or 'function' words (on the basis that they come from open or closed grammatical categories), (ii) have word frequencies of 100 words per million or greater, (iii) are between 3 and 7 letters long, and (iv) the content words are morphologically simple. This yields 40 function words and 60 content words, closely matched for rated imageability, but differing slightly in word frequency and letter length. These content and function words were presented for oral reading together with 20 high imageability filler words (whose purpose was to maintain morale). The third list consists of fifty content words and fifty function words matched exactly for word frequency, in both the Kucera and Francis (1967) and the Thorndike and Lorge (1948) word counts, and for letter length but not matched in terms of imageability. The results on all three lists are shown in table 9.

On Patterson's list, MK is marginally worse at reading function words than content words, but the effect does not reach statistical significance (Fisher exact, $z = 1.17$, $p = .12$). On the lists matched for imageability range, there is no difference between function words and content words, and this result is replicated on the third list.

Finally, we presented MK with the list of nouns and verbs matched for imageability, frequency and length described by Allport and Funnell (1981).

Table 9
Oral word reading—the effects of word class
(i) **List of 'content' and 'function' words from Patterson (1979)**

	N	Proportion correct
'Function words'	60	.85
'Content words'	60	.93

(Fisher exact test, z = 1.17, p > .2)

(ii) **List of 'content' and 'function' words matched approximately for imageability (for details see text)**

	N	Proportion correct	Examples
'Function words'	40	.83	BOTH, OVER
'Content words'	60	.85	KEEP, REASON

(iii) **List of 'content' and 'function' words matched exactly for word frequency and letter length**

	N	Proportion correct	Examples
'Function words'	50	.94	DID, US, EVER
'Content words'	50	.91	MAN, GO, NEED

(iv) **List of matched nouns and verbs, from Allport and Funnell (1981)**

	N	Proportion correct	Examples
Nouns	30	.83	FAITH, FUND
Verbs	30	.93	SERVE, WEAR

Again there was no significant difference in oral word reading as a function of word type.

Summary of MK's performance on oral word reading tasks

In oral word reading MK closely resembles patients described as surface dyslexic (see Patterson, Marshall, and Coltheart 1985). His ability to read nonwords and his tendency to produce phonologically plausible but incorrect readings for irregularly spelled words indicates that he is able to use a SLRR. The occurrence of misreadings on nonwords, especially when they are longer, suggests that this routine is not operating flawlessly. Since he is often able to read an irregular word correctly, it is clear that lexical reading is not entirely abolished. His word reading is not affected by a word's grammatical category or its imageability.

However, these data alone do not indicate whether MK uses a semantic or nonsemantic routine in lexically mediated reading. Because the majority of the words in the lists that we used were regularly spelled, MK might have been generating the appropriate phonology by the SLRR when the routes to addressed phonology failed. Two conclusions are, however, safe:

(i) The SLRR is operating reasonably well (as shown by good nonword reading and phonologically plausible errors in reading real words).

(ii) MK is often able to retrieve addressed phonology for real words (as shown by 50% + accuracy in oral reading of irregular words).

Chapter 4
Visual Lexical Decision

On Coltheart's (1980a) 'easy lexical decision', which involves discriminating short frequent concrete words (e.g., CAR, SCHOOL) from corresponding nonwords (e.g., CAG, SCHOOM), MK scored 49/50 correct. On a more searching task devised by Rickard (1986) involving lexical decision on a set of words varying in rated imageability and rated familiarity MK scored 467/480 correct (see table 10); his hit rate was 0.97 (normal controls, mean 0.99, range 0.94–1.0) and his false positive rate 0.02 (normals, mean 0.01, range 0.02–0.00; control data from Rickard 1986). Clearly he is able to identify real words that are presented in a written form as well as normal controls can. There are two ways in which MK might be performing this task. He could do it by accessing directly entries in an orthographic input lexicon; it would, alternatively, be possible to perform correctly in these lexical decision tasks by sublexical assembly of the stimulus word's phonology and then judging whether the phonological string corresponds to a real word. In this case visual lexical decision might be done on the basis of information in an auditory input lexicon.

If his lexical decision depends on prior phonological recoding via a SLRR, then two types of stimuli should cause problems: phonological recoding is likely to cause him to miss many more irregular words than matched regular words, and to make more false positive errors to pseudo-homophones (e.g., BOTE, PHOCKS) than to matched control nonwords. At least one other surface dyslexic patient, who has been tested in lexical decision with irregular words and pseudo-homophones, performed significantly less well on these words than with regular words and control nonwords, thus indicating some reliance on phonological recoding in visual lexical decision (Kay and Patterson 1985).

MK was presented for lexical decision with 39 regular and 39 irregular words (from Coltheart, Besner, Jonasson, and Davelaar 1979) together with 39 pseudo-homophones and 39 control nonwords matched item by item for word length, and by list for 'N-ness' (the number of real words that can be made by changing each letter of each nonword—a general measure of their visual similarity to real words). Stimuli were presented in random order on a VDU screen and remained in view until MK pressed a key with

Table 10
Visual lexical decision performance as a function of word imageability and familiarity: probability of miss on real word stimuli (number of items in cell in parentheses; stimulus set from Rickard, 1986)

| | Word imageability | | | | |
	Very low	Low	Medium	High	Mean
Familiarity					
Low	.20 (20)	.00 (20)	.00 (15)	—	.07 (55)
Medium	.20 (15)	.05 (20)	.00 (20)	.00 (20)	.05 (75)
High	.00 (20)	.00 (30)	.00 (20)	.00 (20)	.00 (90)
Mean	.13 (55)	.01 (70)	.00 (55)	.00 (40)	

'Extra function words' .00 (20) Nonwords (false positives) .02 (240)

Table 11
Lexical decision with written words: performance with irregular words and pseudohomophones

	Regular words	Irregular words	Pseudo-homophones	Control nonwords
Examples	SPEND	PROVE	CHUZE	THUZE
	TAKE	COME	KORD	KORP
	n = 39	n = 39	n = 39	n = 39
Probability of error	0.00	0.05	0.05	0.00
Mean correct RT (secs)	2.04	2.13	1.96	1.74
(standard deviation)	(1.09)	(0.88)	(0.97)	(0.86)

either left or right hand to indicate his response; latencies were measured from the stimulus onset to the key press.

The results (table 11) shows no significant disadvantage for either pseudohomophones compared to control nonwords or for irregular words compared to regular words. His responses are very slow relative to those of normal subjects in psychological experiments (who are mostly less than 25 years old); they are much less slow in relation to aphasic subjects of his age. We do not attach too much significance to his reaction times, as the instructions did not put any emphasis on speed of response. It is clear that MK does not rely on phonological recoding in visual lexical decision, and his good performance in the Rickard lexical decision task suggests that MK does not have an impaired visual input lexicon; it is sufficiently intact to support normal visual lexical decision.

Chapter 5
Written Word Comprehension

Understanding a written word requires access to a central semantic representation corresponding to that word. This can be done either by direct semantic access following correct categorization of the written word in a visual input lexicon or on the basis of a phonological code. Where a patient is forced to rely solely on a phonological code for access to semantics, s/he will have difficulty in understanding words with homophones. Given the word MAIN it will not be possible to decide if this means 'the most important' or 'long hair at the back of an animal's neck' because the phonology—/meɪn/—does not distinguish between the meanings. Where, in addition, a patient is forced to use an SLRR to generate the phonological code, s/he will find irregular words difficult to understand because the phonological code (from the SLRR) will often be inappropriate. From the (irregular) word BEAR, a SLRR would probably generate the phonology 'beer'; if comprehension depended only on this phonological code the patient would presumably define it as 'a hop-flavored grain-based fermented drink'. With other irregular words the SLRR-generated phonological code would be uninterpretable; given YACHT this (hypothetical) patient might say 'its not a word—it doesn't mean anything'—an appropriate description for the phonological form '/jætʃt/'.

Word to picture matching

MK was tested on the Peabody Picture Vocabulary Test (Dunn 1965). He scored 123/150 with written word presentation (according to the American norms, 111 is the score of an average 18-year-old). With spoken word presentation his score was 113/150, which is significantly worse than with written word presentation (although not severely impaired).

Synonym judgments

One limitation of word-to-picture matching tasks as a method of testing word comprehension is that they are most appropriate for testing of comprehension of picturable, and therefore relatively concrete, words. We therefore tested MK with Coltheart's (1980a) lists of high and low image-ability word pairs for synonym judgments. In this task the patient has to decide whether a pair of written words are very similar in meaning (e.g., CROP—HARVEST; REALITY—TRUTH), or are unrelated (CROP—BAG; REALITY—SARCASM). With pairs of written words, MK was correct on 37/38 judgments with high imageability words, and 34/38 with low imageability words (chance is 19/38). With pairs of spoken words he was worse: 33/38 high imageability and 26/38 low imageability. There is clearly an imageability effect with auditory presentation (Fisher exact, $z = 1.64$, $p = .05$; 95% confidence interval of the accuracy difference is .37 to .001). With written words there is no significant imageability effect ($z = 0.92$, ns); but a real effect might be masked by ceiling effects (the 95% confidence interval for the true difference is .19 to $-.03$).

Definition of high and low imageability written words

MK was presented with the lists of 100 low imageability words matched to 100 high imageability words (described previously for oral reading) for spoken definition; for our convenience in recording his responses he was encouraged to limit them to one or two words. As we were interested in whether MK had accessed the meaning of the appropriate word, rather than how detailed the meaning description that he had accessed was, we ac-cepted as correct anything indicating that MK had some knowledge of the meaning of the word. We would, for example, accept responses of any of the following kinds:

synonym	e.g., FAULT	→ 'mistake'
superordinate	e.g., NOSE	→ 'face'
co-ordinate	e.g., FATHER	→ 'mother'
property	e.g., SUMMER	→ 'hot'
associate	e.g., DEBATE	→ 'Thatcher'

He was correct with 99/100 high imageability words and 67/100 low imageability words. Most of his errors on the low imageability words were vaguely related to the target (e.g., WAIT → 'slow', MERCY → 'tomb') or bore no discernable relationship to the presented word (MATURE → 'shadow', TYPE → 'rodeo'). His difficulty in defining low imageability words may in part be attributable to the fact that abstract words are harder to define; this would account for vague but arguably appropriate responses. This does not, however, account for totally unrelated responses, which occur exclu-sively with low imageability words. It is likely, then, that MK has a genuine problem in understanding written low imageability words.

Picture name judgment

Our definition task only requires partial semantics. To produce the response 'face' to the written word NOSE, for instance, does not require MK to have a meaning representation that can discriminate between NOSE, MOUTH, EAR or any other part of the face. We therefore devised a task which would require more accurate access to the semantics of concrete words.

MK was presented with a picture, and asked to judge whether a written word was the correct name for the picture. Each picture was presented four times; once it occurred with the correct name (e.g., KNEE), once with a close semantic distractor (e.g., ELBOW), once with a phonologically similar real word (which differed from the correct name by a single phoneme; e.g., SEA), and once with a phonologically similar nonword (also differing by a single phoneme from the correct name; e.g., GEE). Because this test was originally devised for auditory presentation, the distractors are defined in terms of auditory similarity; however because (in English) phonologically similar words and nonwords are also orthographically similar, the distractors will give some estimate of the rate of occurrence of the orthographic misperceptions responsible for errors in comprehension. The pictures were 97 items from the '100 picture naming test', excluding 3 items where there is no phonologically similar real word neighbor. The pictures were presented four times in the same order in separate sessions; equal numbers of stimuli of each type occurred in each list, and the order of stimulus types for each item across lists was randomized.

The results are shown in table 12. MK is extremely good at accepting the correct names, and rejecting the two types of phonologically related distractors. With he semantic distractors he (incorrectly) accepts 20% of the items. Thus, for example, he judges that LOBSTER is the correct name for a picture of a CRAB, BRIDLE for SADDLE, SNAKE for WORM, and WIGWAM for TENT. With concrete, picturable words, MK seems to access a semantic representation that is sufficiently elaborated to perform well on tasks that require relatively broad semantic distinctions (as in word-to-picture matching, or

Table 12
Judging the appropriate names for pictures (written word presentation; 97 pictures, chance = .5)

		Response 'Yes'	'No'
Correct name	e.g. KNEE	97	0
Semantically related	e.g. ELBOW	19	78
Phonologically related real word	e.g. SEA	1	96
Phonologically related nonword	e.g. GEE	1	96
Overall proportion correct judgments .95			

word definition); but he has some difficulty when forced to make fine semantic distinctions of the sort required in this task.

These errors could be due to a difficulty in comprehension of the words, or a difficulty in comprehension of the pictures (or both). We will defer our discussion of picture recognition processes until the section on picture naming. There we will argue that MK has no difficulty in picture recognition, and his errors in this name judgment task therefore reflect a genuine but subtle impairment in concrete written word comprehension.

Defining written words with homophones

The four previous tests show that MK performs reasonably well in understanding written words, at least where they are highly imageable. Although he is consistently better at comprehending written words than spoken ones, it is possible that this discrepancy could be explained by some peripheral problem in auditory speech perception. To establish whether he is relying on phonological recoding in written word comprehension, the crucial test is whether he can define words with homophones correctly. If he is phonologically recoding via a SLRR he should only make homophone errors in definition of regular words (because with only regular words will the SLRR yield a definable phonological string); if phonological recoding depends on a lexical route to phonology, he will make homophone errors on both regular and irregular words with homophones.

He was given 25 regular and 25 irregular words with homophones to define; they were presented in two separate sessions, so they only one member of a homophone pair occurred in any one session. There were only four unacceptable definitions:

AIL   → 'petrol, oil is it?'
KNOWS → 'all my words'
KNOW → 'talking'
NONE → 'again'

None of these incorrect definitions could possibly be construed as being definitions of the stimulus word's homophone. This, together with the fact that he was able to define the other 46 words, is strong evidence that he is able to understand written words correctly without having to rely on prior phonological recoding.

Defining regular and irregular written words

As MK is worse at reading aloud irregular words than regular ones, he should be bad at defining irregular words if he relies on phonological recoding in this task. He was therefore presented with the Parkin (1982)

Table 13
The effects of spelling regularity on word definition, and oral word reading (word sets from Parkin, 1982)

	Regular words $n = 33$	Mildly irregular words $n = 33$	Very irregular words $n = 33$
Written word definition	0.94	0.91	0.88
Oral word reading	0.91	0.82	0.52

Table 14
Performance with pseudo-homophones ($n = 80$)

	Proportion correct
Written pseudohomophone definition	0.38
Oral reading of pseudohomophone	0.83
Written real word definition	0.89
Spoken real word definition	0.30

word lists for definition. The results (table 13) show that in definition there is no effect of the stimulus words' regularity, even though he is very much worse at reading irregular words aloud. It is clear that he can easily define written words that he cannot pronounce—he defines very irregular words very much better than he pronounces them (McNemar, $p < .01$).

Defining written pseudo-homophones

The previous two tasks examine MK's performance in word definition where reliance on phonological recoding would cause errors; in this experiment we examine MK's performance in defining pseudo-homophones— a task that *requires* phonological recoding. MK was given 80 pseudo-homophones (e.g., BOTE, PHITE) for definition; in separate sessions he was also given the pseudo-homophones for reading aloud and the corresponding real words (BOAT, FIGHT) in both written and spoken form for definition.

The results are shown in table 14. In pseudo-homophone definition MK is 38% correct. With the corresponding written real words he performs very much better (89% correct). His difficulty with the pseudo-homophones cannot be due to any difficulty in attaining a phonological code—he reads 83% of them aloud correctly. His difficulty appears to lie in accessing semantics from a heard word—he is only 30% correct at defining the spoken words.

The results of this experiment confirm our earlier contention that MK's written word comprehension does not depend on prior phonological recoding: in pseudo-homophone comprehension, which requires phonological recoding, MK performs much worse than in understanding real written words. In an earlier paper we analyzed MK's performance with pseudo-homophones in much greater detail (Howard and Franklin 1987). We showed that his ability to read pseudo-homophones aloud correctly is a function of their length, but definition is independent of length but depends on the visual similarity between the pseudo-homophone and the corresponding real word. On these grounds we argued that MK has to rely on 'approximate visual access' (cf. Saffran and Marin 1977) to comprehend pseudo-homophones and that phonological recoding probably played no role.

Summary of written word comprehension tasks

MK's performance in written word comprehension tasks is generally good, where the stimuli are concrete, but with abstract words his performance is impaired. A more detailed analysis is given in Howard and Franklin (1987).

Compared to previous reports of 'surface dyslexic' patients, MK shows a unique pattern of written word comprehension: there is no evidence that MK ever relies on phonological recoding prior to lexical or semantic access. There are four lines of evidence for this claim:

(i) Comprehension of irregular words is not impaired relative to comprehension of regular words, although reading of irregular words is much worse than the reading of regular words.

(ii) Homophone comprehension errors do not occur with regular or irregular words.

(iii) Lexical decision shows no evidence of effects of phonological recoding—performance is good both with irregular real words and pseudo-homophones.

(iv) Defining real words (which do not have to be phonologically recoded) is very much better than defining pseudo-homophones (which do have to be phonologically recoded).

MK's written word comprehension can be summarized by saying that he pays no attention to the phonological code he creates from a word—given the word MOVE he said 'to go—/məʊv/'.

Chapter 6
Auditory Word Comprehension

Auditory phoneme discrimination

Intact speech-sound perception is necessary for comprehension of the spoken word. At the most peripheral level, a conductive deafness can result in a severe auditory comprehension problem. As we discussed in the introduction, a number of researchers from Goldstein (1906, 1948) onward have suggested that a more central problem in speech sound discrimination might underlie the auditory comprehension difficulties of 'Wernicke's aphasics' and 'word deaf' patients (see Luria 1947).

Pure tone audiometry showed that MK had a 5–20dB hearing loss in both ears across the frequency range 250–8000Hz. This is a normal audiogram for a man of his age.

We tested MK's ability in phoneme discrimination in four different ways. For the first test we assembled a set of 54 pairs of pictures where the names differed in a single phoneme, which was, in all cases, word final (e.g., CALF/CARVE; CAP/CAT). He was presented, on two separate occasions, with the picture pairs and asked to point to the picture whose name was spoken by the examiner; each picture served as the target in one session. The second test was a same/different judgment task involving the picture names from the first test. MK was presented with pairs of spoken words half of which were identical (e.g., 'cat—cat'), and half of which differed only in the final phoneme ('calf—carve'), and asked to judge whether they were the same or different. The third task was an equivalent test in same/different judgments involving pairs of nonwords; the nonwords were generated by changing the initial phoneme of the real words in the previous task (e.g., '/paf—pav/'). In the fourth task the nonwords were reversed so that they differed only in the initial phoneme ('/fap—vap/').

The results (table 15) show that MK is 89–97% correct across the four tasks, even though all four tasks require discrimination of a difference in a single phoneme. While there are no norms for these tests, this level of accuracy would seem adequate for word comprehension.

Table 15
Auditory phoneme discrimination: minimal pair judgments (in each test chance = .50)

	N	Proportion correct
(i) Word to picture matching (word final)	54	.89
(ii) Word minimal pairs (word final)	108	.96
(iii) Nonword minimal pairs (word final)	108	.97
(iv) Nonword minimal pairs (word initial)	108	.91

Auditory rhyme judgments

MK was given 60 pairs of words and asked to judge if they rhymed. Half of the rhyming pairs were orthographic rhymes (e.g., CREAM TEAM) and half were not (COME SUM). Similarly half of the nonrhyming pairs were orthographically similar (FOOT BOOT) and half were not (SHOUT LOOT). MK made 58/60 correct judgments; his two errors were on rhyming pairs that were orthographically dissimilar. The results of this test support the view that MK has access to a good auditory code.

Investigation of MK's short term memory performance, which we report in detail in Howard and Franklin (1989), shows that MK can hold a list of at least four digits in an auditory (and prelexical) input store. This supports the view that he can generate and hold auditory input representations.

Auditory lexical decision

MK was presented the full set of words and nonwords from Rickard's (1986) lexical decision test in spoken form for lexical decision.

Overall MK made 85% correct decisions, which is very much better than chance (probability of miss .19; FP .13, $d' = 2.00$). However he is significantly worse at lexical decision when it is presented auditorily than with written words (overall 97% correct, $d' = 3.93$). Some of his difficulty with auditory lexical decision may be accounted for in terms of problems in accessing the correct entry in the auditory input lexicon. However, as the results in table 16 show, MK is significantly more likely to miss low imageability than high imageability words (Jonckheere trend test, $z = 63.3$; $p < .0001$), although his performance is not significantly related to the words' rated familiarity ($z < 1$; ns). If MK's difficulties in this task were due *solely* to peripheral problems in auditory perception or in loss of information at the level of the auditory input lexicon, we would expect errors to be independent of a word's imageability, and errors might be concentrated on words of lower frequency/familiarity. In lexical decision MK seems to be influenced by access to a semantic representation corresponding to the

Table 16
Auditory lexical decision performance as a function of word imageability and familiarity: probability of miss on real word stimuli (number of items in cell in parentheses; stimulus set from Rickard, 1986)

| | Word imageability | | | | |
	Very low	Low	Medium	High	Mean
Familiarity					
Low	.15 (20)	.30 (20)	.20 (15)	—	.22 (55)
Medium	.33 (15)	.10 (20)	.05 (20)	.00 (20)	.11 (75)
High	.40 (20)	.17 (30)	.20 (20)	.05 (20)	.20 (90)
Mean	.29 (55)	.19 (70)	.15 (55)	.03 (40)	

'Extra function words' .30 (20) Nonwords (false positives) .13 (240)

word; his difficulty with abstract words in lexical decision must therefore reflect in part a difficulty in accessing the semantics for abstract words, and not only a deficit in the auditory input lexicon or at some more peripheral level of processing. In the next section we test whether this hypothesized problem in access to semantics for auditorily presented abstract words can be confirmed in word comprehension tasks.

Auditory word comprehension tasks

The results of the PPVT and Coltheart's synonym judgments with both auditory and written presentation are given in table 17. On both comprehension tasks MK performs worse with auditory presentation; in the synonym judgments MK performs significantly worse with abstract words than concrete words (Fisher exact test, $z = 1.64$; $p = .05$). While this confirms that MK has a problem in the comprehension of abstract words, the PPVT results suggest that he retains some comprehension of very low frequency words; in this test he manages to select the appropriate picture to match to spoken words including 'sepal', 'cincture', 'lanate', 'scallion' and 'chirography'.[4] Bishop and Byng's (1984) test of 'lexical understanding with visual and semantic distractors' (LUVS) presents target items together with distractors that are semantically or visually similar; some targets occur with distractors that are both semantically and visually similar. In this test MK made no errors with auditory or visual presentation.

For a more demanding test of MK's comprehension of picture names, we used a word-to-picture matching task developed by Janice Kay. In this test

4. The Peabody test involves selecting the appropriate picture from a choice of four. Some of these responses may then be right by chance, but because MK's performance never fell to a chance level, we can be sure that he knew at least some of these words.

Table 17
Performance in four tests of word comprehension with auditory and visual presentation: the Peabody Picture Vocabulary Test (Dunn, 1965); Coltheart's (1980a) synonym judgments test; Kay's word-to-picture matching test; and Shallice's word-to-picture matching test

	Auditory presentation	Visual presentation
Peabody Picture Vocabulary Test (150 items; chance = 0.25)	.75	.82
Synonym judgments		
High imageability	.86	.97
Low imageability	.68	.89
Mean	.77	.93
(38 items in each imageability range; chance = 0.5)		
Word-to-picture matching (Kay) (40 items; chance = 0.20)	.88	.98
Word-to-picture matching (Shallice) (chance = 0.25)		
Concrete words ($n = 30$)	.87	.93
Abstract words ($n = 30$)	.50	.63
Emotional words ($n = 15$)	.53	.67
Total ($n = 75$)	.65	.76

a word has to be matched to one of five pictures: there is the target picture (e.g., SWORD), a close semantic distractor (SHIELD), a more distant semantic distractor (GUN), and two unrelated distractors that are semantically related to each other (ANCHOR, CHAIN). With written word presentation MK scored 39/40; his error was selecting a FINGER (a close semantic distractor) for THUMB. With spoken word presentation he scored 35/40; three of his errors were semantically related (two close, one distant), and two unrelated foils. With one of these MK commented on his error; having selected a FROG to the spoken name 'hosepipe', he said: "I thought it was spider." In this case, misrecognition of the heard word as a phonologically similar real word appears to underlie his selection of a semantically unrelated foil.

Shallice's word-to-picture matching test compares comprehension of concrete words to abstract or emotional ones. As table 17 shows, with visual word presentation MK is better with concrete words than either of the other two types; this difference is significant (chi squared (2) = 8.30; $p < .05$). With auditory presentation his general level of performance is somewhat lower, and he shows the same advantage for concrete words (chi squared (2) = 10.10; $p < .01$).

Table 18
Oral definition of words with auditory or visual presentation
(i) **The effects of word imageability and frequency (20 items in each cell)**

	Auditory presentation	Visual presentation
High frequency, high imageability words	.75	.95
Low frequency, high imageability words	.80	.95
High frequency, low imageability words	.65	.95
Low frequency, low imageability words	.55	.80
Total (80 items)	.69	.91

(ii) **The effects of imageability (100 items in each cell)**

	Auditory presentation	Visual presentation
High imageability words	.67	.99
Low imageability words	.27	.67

Defining spoken words

We presented MK with two different lists of high and low imageability words. These were the word sets matched across word frequency and imageability, and the 100 high imageability words matched to 100 low imageability words. We used the same criteria for correct definition described in the section on reading comprehension.

The results are shown in table 18. In the lists varying frequency and imageability, there is no significant word frequency effect with either auditory or visual word presentation. The effect of word imageability approaches significance with auditory presentation, but not with visual presentation. However, the word sets are small. We cannot be sure whether there are or are not real imageability effects from this data (95% confidence limits for true difference is .37 to − .02 with auditory presentation, and .20 to − .05 with visual presentation).

In the longer lists, MK provided 67/100 appropriate definitions for high imageability words, and 27/100 for low imageability words—a highly significant difference. This effect cannot be wholly attributable to some general difficulty with abstract word definition, because MK is very much better at definition of both sets of words with written word presentation. He therefore has a real difficulty with semantic access for both high and low imageability words with auditory presentation, as well as a difficulty with defining low imageability words with both auditory and visual word presentation.

Most of MK's errors in definition bear no clear relationship to their stimuli (e.g., 'vivid' → 'talk', 'genuine' → 'ankle'); some errors may be vaguely related to the target ('bullet' → 'boxing', 'grow' → 'bank'). There are seven errors where we are confident that MK is defining a word that is phonologically similar to the stimulus item. Six of these errors occur with 'low imageability' words (e.g., 'myth' → 'spinster' (cf. 'miss'); 'series' → 'corn' (cf. 'cereal')); one error occurs with a high imageability word ('winter' → 'pane' (cf. 'window')). There may, of course, be other errors of this kind where we do not have the ingenuity to identify the intermediate item.

Word length effects in definition

In the auditory lexical decision experiment, MK appeared to have some difficulty in accessing the correct word form in an auditory input lexicon, with auditorily presented words. In the experiment on the definition of abstract and concrete words, he sometimes misdefines a word as another phonologically similar word. We should therefore predict that MK's comprehension of a word will depend on its confusability with other phonologically similar words. This in turn will be closely correlated with the word's length: single-syllable words such as 'whale' or 'flock' will have many close neighbors with which they could easily be confused (e.g., 'hail', 'while', 'wade'; or 'lock', 'flick', 'flog'). Three-syllable words (e.g., 'crocodile', 'paradise') have few or no real words that differ in only a single phoneme (e.g., 'crocodile' has no neighbors, and 'paradigm' is the only neighbor for 'paradise'). We should therefore predict that MK's comprehension should be better for longer than shorter auditorily presented words.

We therefore presented him with a set made up of 30 words of 1, 2, or 3 syllables. They were closely matched for word frequency and word imageability, and they consisted mostly of relatively high imageability words (for the matching data see appendix 1). They were presented, in random order, in separate sessions for definition in written and spoken form.

The results are shown in table 19. With written word presentation, MK's definition accuracy is consistently high, and there are no effects of word length. With spoken word presentation, on the other hand, there is a highly significant effect of word syllable length (Jonckheere trend test, $z = 2.55$, $p < .01$).

Table 19
The effects of word syllable length in oral word definition (30 items in each cell)

	Auditory presentation	Visual presentation	Examples
One-syllable words	.77	.97	WHALE, FLOCK
Two-syllable words	.90	.93	LEOPARD, MOISTURE
Three-syllable words	.97	.97	CROCODILE, PARADISE

Judgments of picture names

The errors in auditory lexical decision, misdefinitions as phonologically similar words, and the word length effect all point to a problem in word identification at an auditory/phonological level that is in turn causing difficulties in word comprehension. Thus far, the evidence that MK has a deficit in access to semantics once the auditory word form has been identified is less clearly established. This experiment was intended to investigate whether he has difficulty in deciding if semantically related, or phonologically related foils are the appropriate names for pictures. If his difficulty lies only in phonological word identification, he might judge that 'pail' or 'zail' were appropriate names for the picture of a NAIL. If MK has difficulty in accessing a complete semantic representation from a spoken word, he might decide that 'screw' was an appropriate name. He was therefore presented with a spoken version of the name judgment task that we had used in assessing his written word comprehension. This involved three types of incorrect words: *phonologically related real words*, which differed from the correct name by a single phoneme; *phonologically related nonwords*, which also differed from the target by a single phoneme; *semantically related words*—closely related (but phonologically distinct) contrast co-ordinates; and the *correct* name. The items were drawn from the 100 items of the 100 picture naming test, eliminating three pictures whose names had no phonological neighbors. They were presented over four separate sessions; equal numbers of stimuli of each type occurred in each session, and each picture occurred just once, in the same order, in each session.

The results (table 20; experiment 1) show that MK's performance is equally poor with all three types of foil; he manages to reject only 60% of incorrect names. Both the semantically related and the phonologically related names cause him to make errors. If MK's difficulty with the phonological foils resulted from problems in phoneme identification, we would expect him to have particular difficulty with foils which are *phonetically* close to the target. We therefore conducted a *post hoc* analysis, comparing his performance on foils that differ from the target in 1, 2, or 3 of the phonetic features of voicing, manner, and place of articulation. The effect of phonetic similarity does not approach statistical significance with either real word foils (Jonckheere trend test, $z = 0.44$, $p > .3$) or nonword foils ($z = 0.73$, $p > .2$). This confirms our earlier conclusions from the phoneme identification tasks; MK's difficulty lies not in faulty analysis of auditory input but in incorrect word identification in the auditory input lexicon.

Given that MK accepts precisely equal proportions of foils of all three types in the name acceptability judgment task, it is conceivable that MK simply tends to accept incorrect names. In signal detection terms, his

Table 20
Judging the appropriate names for pictures (auditory presentation; 97 pictures, chance = .5)
Experiment 1

		Response	
		'Yes'	'No'
Correct name	e.g. 'knee'	94	3
Semantically related	e.g. 'elbow'	39	58
Phonologically related real word	e.g. 'sea'	39	58
Phonologically related nonword	e.g. '/gi/'	39	58
Overall proportion correct judgments .69			

Effect of phonetic similarity to the target on performance with phonologically related real words and nonwords

No. of distinctive	Real words		Nonwords	
features different	'Yes'	'No'	'Yes'	'No'
1	18	19	19	26
2	10	26	15	17
3	11	13	5	15

Experiment 2

		Response	
		'Yes'	'No'
Correct name	e.g. 'knee'	94	3
Unrelated name	e.g. 'egg'	2	95
Overall proportion correct judgments .97			

problem would be only one of eccentric criterion setting. We therefore ran a second control experiment contrasting his performance on correct names and foils that were neither semantically nor phonologically related to the target. The results can be seen as experiment 2 in table 20. His performance is much improved compared to experiment 1; the false positive rate on unrelated foils is only 2%, compared with 40% in experiment 1. In experiment 2, d' is 3.94, compared with 2.13 in experiment 1. This control experiment therefore establishes that MK has real difficulty in deciding both if phonologically related words and semantically related words are correct picture names.

Conclusions on auditory word comprehension

Across all tasks MK performs less well with auditory word presentation than with words that are visually presented. There is, however, a difficulty in abstract word comprehension common to both modalities of presentation. His difficulty with auditorily presented words cannot be plausibly attributed to any defect in sound recognition, first because he manages a reasonable level of performance in auditory minimal pair judgments, and second because his performance in judging whether picture names are appropriate is independent of the phonetic similarity between the foil and the target. Nor can MK's auditory comprehension difficulty be attributed to any across-the-board degradation in the auditory input lexicon: lexical decision is relatively good with concrete words, and errors occur preferentially with low imageability words. In both lexical decision and auditory definition, word misrecognition is found most frequently with abstract words. In the picture name judgment task, on the other hand, MK accepts as correct picture names 40% of foils that differ from the correct name by a single phoneme. This suggests that MK's expectation of what he could hear is biasing his recognition of the heard word. Thus evidence from all three tasks implies that there is a strong relationship between semantic representations and the auditory input lexicon. It is clear that MK has difficulties in accessing full semantic representations from auditory presentation. In the name judgment task, he accepts 40% of contrast co-ordinates as correct names, which implies that he often accesses semantic representations that are not sufficiently elaborated to distinguish between closely related members of a class. He does not access an inappropriate but complete semantic representation—if he did, he should often reject correct names. In the discussion we will return to the issue of whether misrecognition of auditorily presented words as other words that are phonologically similar can be best accounted for by a deficit in the auditory input lexicon, a deficit in semantic access processes, or an interaction between the two.

In addition to a specific problem in auditory word recognition, MK has difficulty in accessing semantics. This is particularly marked with abstract words, with both auditory and visual presentation. We demonstrated this in synonym judgments, Shallice's word-to-picture matching, and two word definition tasks. There is an advantage for high imageability words in all four tasks, and in each case the extent of the advantage with auditorily presented words is not significantly greater than the advantage with visually presented words. There is, then, an abstract word comprehension deficit that appears to be independent of the modality of presentation.

Chapter 7
Oral and Written Picture Naming

MK has a semantic problem in comprehension of spoken and written words. Picture naming involves accessing a semantic representation from a picture, and using this central semantic representation to retrieve a spoken name (see Seymour 1979; Beauvois 1982; Morton 1985). It therefore obligatorily involves semantic processing.[5] To what extent, then, does MK have a semantic problem in naming that resembles his deficit in word comprehension?

To establish the extent to which MK's naming is disturbed, we presented him with the following three picture naming tests, and asked him, in separate sessions, to produce written and spoken names.

The Graded Naming Test (Warrington and McKenna 1983)

This is a test of relatively rare items: the first picture is a KANGAROO and the last a RETORT. In spoken naming MK scored 11/30. This score is at the lower end of average range for control subjects of MK's age; if minor phonological errors (e.g., PAGODA → '/'pægədə/'; TRAMPOLINE → '/'tæmpəʊlaɪn/', where MK must have accessed the correct output word form) are considered acceptable, the score becomes 18/30, which is a good average score. However, this is is probably below his premorbid level. Three types of error account for most of his errors: 8 semantic errors (e.g., PERISCOPE → 'submarine'; TWEEZERS → 'penknife'), 5 phonological errors (e.g., TRAMPOLINE → '/'tæmpəʊlaɪn/'; PAGODA → '/'pægədə/'), and 4 'inflectional/derivational' errors (e.g., BELLOWS → 'bellow').

In written naming of the same set of pictures, MK scored 12/30 correct; again, once (minor) spelling errors are discounted, his score improves

---

5. Kremin (1987) presents evidence that she claims demonstrates that picture naming is possible without semantic mediation. She found two cases of patients who, while performing badly in judging whether pictures were associated, nevertheless could name accurately; we are not convinced that failure in associative judgments demonstrates conclusively that conceptual-semantic representations are impaired—it could equally reflect a deficit in making judgments of this kind.

to 18/30. His errors on written naming were very similar to the ones he made in oral naming; for example: 5 semantic errors (e.g., PERISCOPE → SUBMARINE; LEOTARD → GYMS), 6 spelling errors (e.g., KANGAROO → KINGEROO; TRAMPOLINE → TRAMPLEINE), and 5 'inflectional/derivational' errors (e.g., SCARECROW → CROW).

The Boston Naming Test (Kaplan, Goodglass, and Weintraub 1976).

The Boston Naming Test (BNT) is a rather less demanding test, covering a wider range of difficulty. The first items are BED and TREE, nos. 30 and 31 are HARMONICA and RHINOCEROS, and the final items PROTRACTOR and ABACUS. The sixty test items were presented, omitting the PRETZEL which is unknown in the United Kingdom. In spoken naming MK scored 35/59. He made 8 semantic errors (e.g., UNICORN → 'pegasus'; SEAHORSE → 'fishhorse'), 8 phonological errors (e.g., FUNNEL → 'fennel', COMB → /kɒm/), 3 semantic then phonological errors (e.g., ACCORDION → '/kɒnsɜteɪnd/—cf. [concertina]), 2 inflectional/derivational errors (e.g., TREE → 'trees'), and 3 others.

With written naming MK scored 37/59; there were 9 semantic errors (e.g., UNICORN → PEGASUS; SEAHORSE → FISH OF HORSE), 6 spelling errors (e.g., HELICOPTER → HALICOPTER), 3 semantic then spelling errors (e.g., ACCORDION → CONCERTAIN), 2 inflectional/derivational errors (e.g., TREE → TREES), and 1 other.

On this version of the BNT, a sample of 84 normal subjects had a mean score of 55.7 with a range of 42–60 (Kaplan, Goodglass, and Weintraub 1976); MK's naming level is just below this range, but the control subjects are younger than he is. Proper normative data covering MK's age range is only available for an 85-item enlarged version of the test; Borod, Goodglass, and Kaplan (1980) report a normal cut off score of 47 for 60–69-year-olds (55%). On the 60-item test, MK manages 59% on the spoken version and 63% on the written. On the assumption that the 20 additional items on the BNT cover the whole difficulty range of the test, MK's performance levels are around the bottom end of the normal range as they were on the GNT.

Comprehension of pictures

MK makes semantic errors in naming (e.g., PERISCOPE → 'submarine'). There are three possible explanations (see Butterworth, Howard, and McLoughlin 1984):

(a) on the basis of the picture he retrieves an *incorrect* but complete *semantic representation* (because of misaddressing of semantic representations from the picture recognition system), which he then correctly names.

(b) On the basis of the picture he can retrieve an *underspecified semantic representation*. This specifies a range of semantically related phonological word forms, including the correct one ('submarine', 'periscope', 'torpedo', 'U-boat' ...). The one that is actually produced is a matter of chance, or selection by some nonsemantic criterion (e.g., the most frequent).

(c) He retrieves a full and correct semantic representation, but, due to an *impairment in output from the central semantic system*, he loses some semantic information, so that the semantic specification used to address phonological word forms is underspecified. A variant on this final proposal was advanced by Patterson (1978) as an explanation for semantic errors in reading; she called this account 'response blocking'. She suggests that where phonological word forms cannot be successfully accessed or output (because they are in some way 'blocked'), the patient might relax the semantic specification used for word retrieval to enable some (semantically related) response to be produced. As Morton and Patterson (1980) point out, it may in practice be very difficult to differentiate these variants.

These three types of impairment can be differentiated using a picture judgment task. Consider an item where MK has to match a picture of a KENNEL to a picture of a CAT or a picture of a DOG. If he accesses incorrect semantics, he will make errors in this task; say he attains the conceptual representation [DOG] from the picture of a CAT—he might choose this to go with the KENNEL. If he retrieves underspecified semantics, he might access the representation [SOME KIND OF HOUSEHOLD PET] from both the CAT and DOG picture. He will then have no way of choosing between the two responses. If on the other hand, his difficulty is in output from the semantic system, but the conceptual semantic representations that he accesses are unimpaired, he will be able to perform this kind of task, involving conceptual matching of pictures, normally.

To test his picture recognition abilities, MK was given the three-picture version of the 'Pyramids and Palm Trees' test (Howard and Patterson, unpublished). This consists of matching a picture to one of a pair of coordinate choices on the basis of a semantic association; consistent correct performance is only possible if the pictures are correctly recognized and full semantic information about them is retrieved. For one item, described above, the patient would have to choose between the picture of a DOG and a picture of a CAT to go with a picture of a KENNEL; in another item, a picture of a PALM TREE or a PINE TREE to go with the picture of a PYRAMID. On this test MK scored 52/52, demonstrating that he can retrieve semantic information from pictures.

We should not, however, assume that there is a single conceptual-semantic representation corresponding to a picture. On the basis of neuropsychological evidence a number of authors have argued that there are separable verbal and nonverbal semantic systems (e.g., Warrington 1975; Beauvois 1982; Shallice 1987). One could then distinguish between impairments to the verbal semantic system, the nonverbal semantic system, and the transmission of information between them; this last type of impairment is what Beauvois (1982) describes as 'optic aphasia'. To distinguish these, there are two further versions of the 'Pyramids and Palm Trees' test. In the three-word version, the picture triads are replaced by the written picture names; so, for example, a patient might have to match the word KENNEL to either the word DOG or the word CAT. The third version involves matching a written word to one of two pictures. A patient with defective visual word recognition or a defective verbal semantic system should have difficulty with the three-written-word version. A patient who had specific difficulty in tasks involving coordination of verbal and nonverbal conceptual knowledge (i.e., an 'optic aphasic') might perform well in the three-word version and the three-picture version, but might have difficulty in the word-to-picture version. MK, however, had no difficulty with either of these versions; he scored 52/52 on both tests.

In line with our earlier results demonstrating that MK has difficulties in auditory word comprehension, he does make errors in two versions of the 'Pyramids and Palm Trees' test that involve the comprehension of spoken words. In matching a spoken word to one of two pictures, he scores 48/52, and in matching a spoken word to one of two written words, he scores 45/52.

He was asked to name aloud all 156 pictures from the test, presented in their original triads. He named 115/156 correctly. His errors on the remainder were overwhelmingly semantically related. For example he named SHEEP as 'cows', BOOTS as 'shoes', SPIDER as 'scorpion', BED as 'cot'. In matching pictures, MK had successfully chosen a BUTTERFLY rather than a DRAGONFLY to go with a CATERPILLAR. When naming them, though, he called the CATERPILLAR a 'slug' and the DRAGONFLY a 'gnat'.

MK's semantic errors in picture naming do not reflect degraded semantic representations, as he is able to perform normal semantic judgments on these pictures. We are therefore confident that MK's naming errors reflect a defect in *output* from the semantic system; his semantic representations for concrete, picturable items are intact, or at least much more intact than is reflected by the naming responses he makes. Patterson's 'response blocking' theory will probably not account for these data. His naming scores are very close to normal; therefore few items can be 'blocked'. As a result we would expect his semantic errors to be very closely related to the targets. However, quite distant errors are common; for example CANDLE → 'flame', TWEEZERS → 'penknife'. This suggests that MK's problem is more likely to be accounted for by loss of information in output from the semantic system, rather than blocked entries in an output lexicon.

The 100 picture naming test

MK was presented with 100 pictures from the set of 'Cambridge pictures' (Patterson, Purell, and Morton 1983). These are pictures for which at least 90% of normal subjects produce the same name. The 100 items were selected from the pictures whose names occur in the MRC Psycholinguistic Database (Coltheart 1981) with values for the following: word frequency from the Thorndike and Lorge (1948) and Kucera and Francis (1967) counts; rated familiarity, imageability, and concreteness; rated age of acquisition and word length, in terms of the number of phonemes in the word and the number of letters. In spoken naming MK scored 82/100. There were 14 semantic errors (e.g., PENCIL → 'pen'; SKIRT → 'dress'; ARCH → 'church'), 2 phonologically related errors, 1 suffix error, and 1 other. In written naming he scored 77/100. He made 19 semantic errors (e.g., PYRAMID → SPHINX; SKIRT → DRESS; ARCH → CHURCH), and 4 spelling errors. This level of performance is clearly defective; Davis (1987) showed that 13 normal controls made two errors or less in naming these 100 pictures. The effects of all eight variables on MK's performance in spoken or written naming were investigated in multiple *t*-tests; in spoken naming, no variable had an effect that approached statistical significance. With written naming, there was a significant effect of word length when measured either as phoneme length ($t(98) = 2.43$, $p = .028$) or word letter length ($t(98) = 1.99$, $p = .049$). As one might expect, these two variables are strongly correlated ($r = 0.80$); as a result it is impossible to sort out statistically which variable is responsible for the effect; since, however, the task is written naming, we suspect on logical grounds that the relevant variable is word letter length. It is clear that MK is significantly worse at written naming of pictures with longer names.

His performance in spoken naming is closely related to his performance in written naming; MK writes correctly 89% of names produced orally and only 22% of those not named correctly. This degree of consistency is highly significant (contingency coefficient $C = .510$, $p < .001$). MK's written naming therefore resembles his spoken naming not only in the types of errors and their relative frequencies but also in the items that attract errors.

Naming pictures with irregularly spelled names

We noticed that, when asked to name a picture whose name had an irregular spelling-to-sound correspondence (e.g., 'bear'), MK would occasionally produce an error that corresponded to the 'regularized' form of that word (e.g., 'beer'). Interpretation of these errors is not entirely straightforward; MK does make occasional output phonological errors, and some of these errors with irregular words could, by chance, correspond to the 'phonologically plausible' form of that word; that is, they would be, in an extension of Butterworth's (1979) terminology, 'jargon regularizations'. We therefore assembled two sets of pictures that had names with an irregular spelling-to-sound relation. He was given the pictures for oral naming and their written names for oral word reading. On the first set of 20 pictures (compiled by Sally Byng and Max Coltheart), 15 were named correctly; the 5 naming errors were as follows:

2 Multiword	MONEY	→ 'monkey, pounds, cash'
responses	FOOT	→ 'shoes, little ankles, soles'
3 Phonologically	COMB	→ '/kɒmb/'
plausible errors	BEAR	→ '/bɪə/'
	CANOE	→ '/kænəʊ/'

In oral reading of these names MK also made 5 errors:

4 Phonologically	COMB	→ '/kəʊmb/'
plausible errors	BEAR	→ '/bɪə/'
	PEAR	→ '/pɪə/'
	BOWL	→ '/baʊl/'
1 other error	LEOPARD	→ '/lɛməd/'

Since phonologically plausible errors make up three of MK's errors in oral naming of these pictures, it is unlikely that they are chance occurrences. MK does, on some occasions, (mis)use orthographic information in generating an oral naming response.

To confirm the existence of orthograhically based errors in oral naming, we presented MK with a further set of 45 pictures with irregularly spelled names (there is partial overlap between the two sets). In oral naming MK made four errors:

2 Phonologically	COMB	→ '/kəʊmb, kɒm/'
plausible errors	SEWING	→ '/su/ machine'
	MACHINE	
2 other errors	SCISSORS	→ 'scissor'
	BLOUSE	→ 'smocks, /pɪə'nəʊfə/' [cf. 'pinafore'].

In oral reading of these 45 picture names MK made 7 errors:

6 Phonologically	COMB	→ '/kɒmb/'
plausible errors	BEAR	→ '/bɪə/'
	ACORN	→ '/ə'kɔn/'
	HEART	→ '/hɜt/'
	SEWING	→ '/'suɪŋ/ machine'
	MACHINE	
	TRIANGLE	→ '/tri'æŋgəl/'
1 other error	RAZOR	→ '/'raɪzə/'.

Again, with irregularly spelled words, the majority of MK's errors in oral naming that are phonologically related to the target are phonologically plausible renderings of the orthography of the word.

The extent to which he does this is difficult to determine. Overall these types of errors are fairly rare; however, (a) very exceptional words are quite unusual in the corpus of picture names, and (b) MK makes relatively few errors on reading irregular words (particularly, as we shall show, with concrete words). Thus there could be instances where MK is 'reading' the picture name internally but is reading it correctly so it is indistinguishable from direct picture naming.

Conclusions from the naming tasks

On standardized naming tests MK manages scores that are around the bottom of the normal range; his naming is almost certainly below his premorbid level but not severely disturbed, at least with concrete, picturable items. We know of no way in which we can systematically test his word *retrieval* for abstract words, given that his auditory and visual abstract word *comprehension* is disturbed and, as we document elsewhere, his sentence comprehension is very limited (Howard and Franklin 1989). However, in word definition tasks MK produces (appropriately) an impressive range of abstract words. This includes:

quiet	→ 'mute'		mature	→ 'ancient'
myth	→ 'fable'		theory	→ 'method'
blonde	→ 'ashen'		toil	→ 'labour'
tongue	→ 'labial'		tweezers	→ 'pincher'

Low frequency concrete words are also common:

golf	→ 'niblick'		queen	→ 'regent'
meadow	→ 'lea'		silver	→ 'platinum'
knife	→ 'stiletto'		manage	→ 'bureau'
bomb	→ 'howitzer'		market	→ 'bazaar'
foam	→ 'hydrant'		ghost	→ 'spectre'
village	→ 'hamlet'		porch	→ 'portico'
chocolate	→ 'bonbon'		paradise	→ 'Eden'

On this basis we are inclined to believe that MK's word retrieval abilities are not severely disturbed for abstract words; but this is a suspicion that we have no means to confirm.

Yet, although we do not think that MK's word retrieval problem is quantitatively severe, we have qualitative evidence of its nature. His performance in the 'Pyramids and Palm Trees' test indicates that his ability to access the semantics of (concrete) words and pictures is reasonably intact;

nevertheless he makes a substantial number of semantic errors in naming, which must reflect a breakdown in *output* from the semantic system. There is a striking similarity between his performance in spoken and written naming in three different ways. Not only are levels of performance in the two tasks very similar, but he also produces very similar error responses in the two tasks; and there is consistency between the tasks—the same items attract errors in oral and written naming. This similarity suggests that there is a common underlying locus of impairment; in the last section of this book we will return to the issue of whether impairment to a single output process from the semantic system could account for this pattern of impairment.

MK is a 'surface dyslexic' in reading. His written naming performance indicates that he is not 'surface dysgraphic', at least not in written naming. Curiously, investigators of patients who show phonological spelling have neglected to report on written naming, concentrating instead on writing to dictation (possibly because like Hatfield and Patterson's (1983) patient TP the anomia is so severe that useful data cannot be gathered). Where surface dysgraphic patients rely upon a sublexical routine for generating written word responses, they should make phonologically plausible spelling errors in written naming. We could find written naming results for only one surface dysgraphic person: HAM, a French patient reported by Kremin (1985), named a key, CLÉ as CLAI, VERRE → VERT and SCIE → SIE. All of these are 'phonologically plausible errors' in French. There is no evidence that MK makes errors of this kind in written naming (or, as we shall demonstrate below, in writing to dictation); he is therefore a surface dyslexic who is not a surface dysgraphic.

While MK does not appear to make phonologically based errors in *written* naming, he does sometimes make errors in *spoken* naming that incorporate orthographic information about the name. He, for example, both reads the word COMB and names the picture of a COMB as '/kɒmb/'; the only plausible source for the word final /b/ in spoken naming is the spelling. It is unlikely that these errors can be explained as phonological errors that just happen to resemble the orthography: first, with pictures whose names have an irregular spelling-to-sound correspondence, orthographically based errors are much more frequent than other nonorthographic phonologically related errors; second, some kinds of errors occur *only* where they have a source in the orthography—we can, for example, find no examples of insertion of word final /b/ that is not present in the spelling. This is, as far as we are aware, the first demonstration of orthographically based errors in oral naming; we will return in the final section to the implications this has for lexical information processing routines.

Chapter 8
Effects of Imageability and Strategy in
Irregular Word Reading

MK's overall level of performance in oral naming of pictures is only mildly impaired. The word comprehension tasks reported above indicate that he has better access to semantics for high imageability written words than for low imageability words. With high imageability words, a semantic reading routine is likely to yield reasonably accurate information—he can both access the appropriate area in the semantic system from written words and use a semantic representation to access a phonological word form. With low imageability words, on the other hand, the semantic reading routine is impaired, because of his difficulties in comprehension of visually presented low imageability words. Even with concrete words the semantic reading routine is not working perfectly. In the task of judging the appropriate written names for pictures, MK accepted 20% of close semantic distractors. If he were to rely solely on a semantic routine for word reading, we should predict that he would make semantic errors in concrete word reading and be better at reading concrete words than abstract ones.

Many theorists have argued that there is a lexical but nonsemantic direct route from a visual input lexicon to a phonological output lexicon (e.g., Schwartz, Saffran, and Marin 1980; Funnell 1983a; Coltheart 1985). If MK had a routine of this kind, he would be able to read all familiar, real words—which he cannot. This direct route cannot, therefore, be intact. The third routine available for reading—the SLRR—must be broadly intact; MK is able to read short nonwords with considerable accuracy, and the majority of his reading errors with irregular words reflect the operation of a route of this kind.

Even if the semantic reading routine is not working perfectly, it might contribute some information in reading. With another 'surface dyslexic' patient, Margolin, Marcel, and Carlson (1985) were able to demonstrate that both phonological and semantic information could contribute partial information to word reading. If the semantic routine does contribute, it will do so most effectively with high imageability words; in consequence, MK will have to rely more on the SLRR with low imageability words. A regularity effect in word reading should therefore be more marked with low imageability than high imageability words.[6]

It is also possible that the use of these two reading routines may be under strategic control. MK may choose between the different reading routines available according to the demands of the task. If by changing the nature of the reading task, we can alter the extent to which his reading of irregular words is impaired, we will have demonstrated that he has two different reading routines available and the allocation of resources between them is under strategic control.

Word regularity and imageability effects in reading

To test the prediction that regularity effects in oral word reading would be more marked with low imageability words, we assembled a list based on information from the MRC Psycholinguistic Database (Coltheart 1981). This consists of 65 high imageability regular words, 65 high imageability irregular words, 55 low imageability regular words, and 55 low imageability irregular words. All four word sets were matched for Kucera and Francis (1967) word frequency, letter length, and phoneme length; within imageability bands, lists were matched for imageability (matching data are given in appendix 1).

The results of oral reading of these word lists are given in table 21. With high imageability words there is a regular word advantage of only 7%; this does not reach statistical significance (Fisher exact test, $z = 1.09$, $p = .14$; 95% confidence interval for regular word advantage -3% to 19%); with low imageability words the advantage for regular words is 24%, which is highly significant ($z = 2.80$, $p = .003$; 95% confidence interval for regular word advantage 9% to 38%).

However, one artifactual account of this interaction can be proposed. In our earlier investigations of regularity effects, we demonstrated that MK was much less accurate on very irregular words than on mildly irregular ones. If the abstract irregular words are 'more' exceptional than the concrete irregular words, then our results would reflect a confounding between imageability and degree of regularity. We know of no satisfactory measure for 'degree of regularity', so we cannot simply demonstrate that the irregular word lists are of equivalent difficulty. We therefore decided to give the same lists to other control surface dyslexics. We considered using real 'surface dyslexic' patients; we rejected this idea because, had they too shown an interaction between regularity and imageability, we would not know whether both they and MK were using a semantic reading route for

---

6. Shallice and Warrington (1980) make exactly this prediction, as a pattern of performance their model would predict but which had never been observed.

Table 21
a. The effects of spelling regularity and word imageability on oral word reading

	Proportion correct			
	High imageability words		Low imageability words	
	Regular	Irregular	Regular	Irregular
	$n = 65$	$n = 65$	$n = 55$	$n = 55$
Examples	EAGLE	WALLET	TREATY	SUBTLE
	RED	SON	MOOD	PUSH
	VINE	VASE	DEAR	LOSE
MK	.92	.85	.91	.67
"Speech"	.87	.22	.75	.25
"Text to speech"	.92	.45	.80	.55

b. Post hoc analysis of the effects of word frequency on oral reading (n is between 10 and 18 in each cell; word frequency from Kucera and Francis (1967))

	Proportion correct			
Word frequency	High imageability words		Low imageability words	
(words/million)	Regular	Irregular	Regular	Irregular
1–8	.89	.67	.94	.47
9–20	.82	.94	1.0	.70
21–60	1.0	.93	.91	.73
61 +	1.0	.88	.82	.81

the more concrete words or whether there was an effect of degree of regularity. We therefore decided to use two control surface dyslexic subjects for which we could be sure that they could not be using semantic information in word reading: we used two cheap word reading programs designed for the BBC microcomputer—'Speech' by Superior Software, and 'Text to Speech' by Computer Concepts. Both of these programs achieve some success in reading irregular words but also make substantial numbers of phonologically plausible errors in reading. Their performance in reading the high and low imageability regular and irregular words is given alongside MK's in table 21. Both programs show highly significant regularity effects with both imageability ranges (Fisher exact, $p < .01$ or better). If anything, both programs show greater advantages for regular words with high imageability compared to the low imageability words—this is the opposite of MK's pattern. The effects with MK, therefore, are unlikely to be attributable to any simple confounding between imageability and degree of regularity.

Our prediction is therefore confirmed; MK is using information from a semantic lexical reading routine in oral reading; it is more likely to yield useful information for high imageability words. Errors in reading irregular words—which reflect reliance on a SLRR—are only a major feature of MK's reading when he is faced with low imageability stimuli.

These data allow us to investigate whether word frequency affects MK's oral word reading. In a *post hoc* analysis whose results are shown in table 21, we found that there were significant effects of word frequency with high and low imageability irregular words, and with low imageability regular words (Jonckheere trend test, $p < .05$ in all three cases), but there was no significant effect with high imageability regular words. Inspection of the results in table 21 shows that this effect is due to poor performance with the words in the very lowest frequency range, 1 to 8 words per million. This demonstration of a word frequency effect in oral word reading should be treated with caution; we have shown that in Parkin's (1982) lists MK's reading is a function of degree of regularity of spelling-to-sound relationship. We have no way of knowing whether degree of regularity is confounded with frequency in these lists. But a word frequency effect in irregular word reading is not surprising; in visual lexical decision MK makes errors only with words of lower rated familiarity (which is in effect words of lower frequency). If some of these low frequency items are missing from his visual input lexicon, he will be unable to read them aloud using a lexical routine. He will therefore be obliged to rely on a SLRR, which will yield incorrect responses with irregular words. That there are more errors in reading irregular words of very low frequency aloud is therefore consistent with his errors with low frequency words in visual lexical decision.

The effects of task context on irregular word reading

The previous experiment demonstrates that, for MK, both the SLRR and the lexical semantic routine are contributing information in oral word reading although neither is operating faultlessly. If the relative contribution of these two routines is under strategic control, we should be able to affect MK's success in oral reading of irregular words by manipulating the context in which they are presented.

We presented MK with a list of 77 highly irregular words for oral reading in the following four conditions:

(a) The irregular words were presented as single words intermixed with 131 nonwords for oral reading.

(b) The irregular words were presented as a list of real words for oral reading.

(c&d) MK was presented with pairs of words; half the pairs were synonyms or near synonyms and half were unrelated. He was asked to judge whether the words were synonyms and then to read the second word aloud. The lists were presented twice so that each of the 77 words occurred once as part of a synonymous pair (condition c) and once in a nonmatching pair (condition d).

Table 22
The effects of list context on oral reading of irregular words ($n = 77$)

	Proportion correct
a. Presented mixed with 131 nonwords	.61
b. Presented as a list of real words	.77
c. Read after 'yes' synonym judgement	.75
d. Read after 'no' synonym judgement	.74

We predicted that the nonword list condition (a) should encourage the use of a SLRR, and as a result irregular word reading should be poor in this condition. The synonym judgments conditions (c&d) require MK to access the meaning corresponding to the presented word prior to producing the reading response, which should encourage him to use a lexical-semantic reading routine; irregular word reading should therefore improve in the synonym judgments conditions relative to the non-word lists. The second, word-only list condition (b) is intended as a neutral control, which corresponds to the conditions under which we normally present real word lists.

The results are shown in table 22. There is a significant difference in correct reading of the irregular words across the four lists (Cochran $Q(3) = 8.12$; $p < .05$). The list presented mixed with nonwords is read significantly less well than either of the other three lists (McNemar's test, $p < .05$ in all three cases). This demonstrates that MK can move resources between a lexical and nonlexical reading routine depending on the demands of the task. With lists of real words, it appears that MK routinely uses as much semantic-lexical information as he has available, as further encouragement to use a semantic routine does not affect his reading accuracy.

Coltheart and Funnell (1987) show that their surface dyslexic subject HG only made significant numbers of errors with words with irregular spelling-to-sound correspondences when they were presented mixed with other nonwords. Like us, they interpret their results in terms of a shift of resources between lexical and sublexical reading routines. With their patient they are unable to exclude a second possibility; this is that HG uses the SLRR to generate a possible phonology, and then decides if it is a possible real word on the basis of whether the phonological string corresponds to an entry in a phonological lexicon. Once nonwords are included in the list, phonological recoding cannot be used as an error-detection strategy. Coltheart and Funnell (1987) argue that HG uses a checking strategy of just this kind in visual lexical decision but not in reading words aloud.

With MK there is no such ambiguity. As we have shown in tasks with pseudo-homophones (see above, and Howard and Franklin 1987), MK cannot decide whether a phonological string generated by his SLRR is a real word or not. Since he does not have this checking procedure available, the differences between accuracy in irregular word reading in different contexts is most plausibly explained as a shift of resources between the lexical and sublexical routines.

Chapter 9
Oral Repetition and Writing to Dictation

In the model of lexical processing we are using, three separate routines can be used for oral repetition of auditorily presented words. A sublexical routine (routine 1 in figure 4) uses the 'subword level auditory-to-phonological conversion' system to convert auditory input codes into output phonology; this routine can be used to repeat both real words and nonwords, by processing them in terms of segments smaller than whole known words. The second, 'direct route' (routine 2 in figure 4) involves a heard word accessing an entry in the auditory input lexicon, which directly addresses an (abstract) specification of the word's spoken form in the phonological output lexicon; this is used to drive the articulatory processes involved in saying the word. As this route involves accessing whole word lexical representations, it can only be used to repeat real words; because it does not involve accessing central semantic representations, its operation should not be sensitive to any semantic factors. The third, 'semantic' repetition routine (routine 3 in figure 4) involves access to semantic representations as an intermediate level of coding. The heard word accesses an entry in the auditory input lexicon which, in turn, addresses a central semantic specification in the cognitive system. This semantic representation is then used to access an entry in the phonological output lexicon. Because in this routine there is a point at which words are coded only in terms of their meaning, a patient relying on this route alone might be expected to make some semantic errors, at least where words have synonyms that can be assumed to share the same meaning representation. We have already established that for MK access to central semantic representations is impaired for low imageability words relative to high imageability words; if he relies exclusively on the semantic routine in repetition, we would expect that high imageability words will be repeated more successfully than low imageability words, and semantic errors should occur.

For writing to dictation the 'logogen model' offers three analogous processing routines. In current versions of the model, however, two are partially parasitic on the corresponding word repetition routines, as they involve using the corresponding repetition routines to access output phonological representations as an intermediate stage in processing. The 'sub-

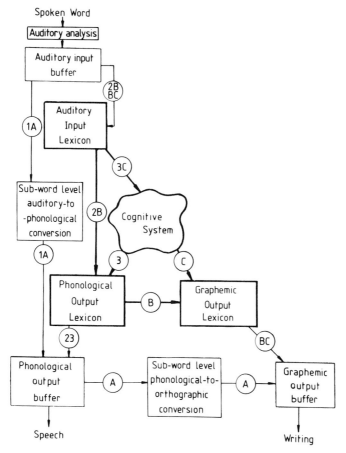

Figure 4
Routines for oral word repetition and writing to spoken dictation. The numbers and letters
in circles on arrows refer to routines using these processes. Oral repetition: (1) sublexical
repetition routine, (2) lexical nonsemantic routine, (3) lexical semantic routine. Writing to
dictation: (A) sublexical routine, (B) lexical nonsemantic routine, (C) lexical semantic routine.

lexical routine' for writing to dictation (routine A in figure 4) involves using the process of 'subword level auditory-to-phonological conversion' to convert the heard word (or nonword) into an output phonological form; the process of 'subword level phonological-to-orthographic conversion' then converts this into an output orthographic code which drives the writing process. This routine can be used to write words and nonwords to dictation, although phonologically plausible spelling errors will occur with real words whose spelling is not unambiguously deducible from their phonology. In contrast, the 'direct routine' for writing to dictation (routine B in figure 4) will work only for familiar real words; as long as the words are fully specified in their lexical representations, it should yield correct responses for all real words.[7] An entry accessed in the auditory input lexicon addresses directly the corresponding entry in the phonological output lexicon; this, in turn, addresses an entry in the orthographic output lexicon that specifies the word's written form. The third 'semantic routine' (routine C in figure 4) involves accessing a central semantic code via an entry in the auditory input lexicon. The semantic representation is used to retrieve an entry in the orthographic output lexicon, which drives the process of producing the written word form. Relying exclusively on this routine for writing to dictation should result in MK making semantic errors, with superior performance with high imageability words compared to that with low imageability words, because of his auditory comprehension impairment for abstract words.

The scheme in figure 4 allows three additional, more complex routes for writing to dictation, which are made up from elements of the other routines. They are omitted from the diagram for reasons of simplicity. They are:

Routine D. AIB → AIL → CS → POL → GOL → GOB. This routine involves semantic mediation, so in a patient using it there might be imageability effects or semantic errors in writing to dictation. Since output goes via the phonological output lexicon, real word homophone errors should occur. The real signature of this routine would be homophone errors superimposed on semantic errors: the response COLONEL when asked to write 'nut', would be strong evidence for the use of this routine.

Routine E. AIB → AIL → CS → POL → POB → (via sub-lexical P-to-O conversion) GOB. Again there is semantic mediation so we might expect imageability effects or semantic errors. Because it depends on a sublexical conversion of orthography to phonology, there will be

7. As Patterson (1986) observes, words with homophones (e.g., 'read'/'reed'), even if they are presented in a disambiguating context, will not be written reliably by this routine, unless there is some semantic influence on the process.

phonologically plausible written responses, which are not necessarily words. One signature of this routine, then, would be phonologically plausible nonword responses superimposed on semantic errors; for example 'boat' written as YOTT.

Routine F. AIB → AIL → (via 'direct route') POL → POB → (via sub-lexical P-to-O conversion) GOB. Since this routine does not involve semantic mediation there should be no semantic errors or effect of imageability. Nonword repetition will be impossible, demonstrating that the patient can only access output phonology lexically; phonologically plausible spelling errors should occur reflecting the use of 'subword level phonological-to-orthographic conversion'. Like all processes involving the lexical, and nonsemantic routines, it will be relatively hard to establish that this routine was being used, as this involves excluding a role for semantic routines.

In this chapter we will present the results of investigations of MK's oral repetition and writing to dictation together. This is because the patterns of performance, and of errors in the two tasks, are strikingly similar; we shall argue that both tasks are performed principally on the basis of 'semantic routines'. First we will investigate the effects on performance of a number of different factors—lexicality (words v. nonwords), word imageability, part of speech, word length, and morphological form; then we will present a slightly more detailed analysis of the types of errors produced and consider some of the factors responsible for production of these errors.

Oral repetition and writing to dictation of nonwords

MK was given 19 monosyllabic nonwords for oral repetition; he repeated none correctly. 17 of his errors were real words. Some were phonologically similar to the nonword—for example '/haɪl/' → 'hale', '/reɪm/' → 'rain', '/faɪd/' → 'fine'; other real word errors bore no obvious relation—for example '/zul/' → 'slight', '/rælb/' → 'little', '/kɪm/' → 'sleep'. The other two errors were:

'/fɪd/'   →   '/fɪŋkɪ/'
'/trɛb/'   →   '/krəmɪən/'.

MK is clearly unable to use a 'sublexical routine' for nonword repetition. We can identify with some precision the point at which this routine is breaking down. Phonemic discrimination in auditorily presented nonwords is not grossly impaired, as he performs minimal pair judgments on nonwords well. Assembly and production of spoken nonwords is not grossly impaired, as he reads single syllable nonwords aloud with reasonable accuracy. For the same reason he cannot be operating some general 'lexical bias' in speech production (cf. Stemberger 1985). His impairment must therefore lie in the process of converting nonword auditory input codes into nonword output phonological codes—that is, the process of 'subword level auditory-to-phonological conversion'.[8]

As described above, the lexical model postulates that writing nonwords to dictation will also require the use of 'subword level auditory-to-phonological conversion'. If, as we have argued, this process is not available for nonword repetition, MK will also be unable to write nonwords to dictation.

MK was given 20 nonwords to write to dictation. As in repetition, he got none correct, and 16 of his errors were real words; some of these were phonologically similar to the target (e.g., '/vɔd/' → BROAD, '/haɪl/' → FILE, '/naɪm/' → KNIFE), but others had no obvious relationship (e.g., '/reɪm/' → GRAPH, '/rælb/' → DRAFT, '/faʊt/' → POINT). The remaining 4 errors were as follows:

'/eɪf/'   → GOOF
'/bɒɪm/'   → GWINE
'/zul/'   → SUBBLSDEY
'/ræld/'   → HERALDO

Clearly MK is unable to repeat nonwords or to write them to dictation. Any success in these tasks with real words will therefore be attributable to his use of one of the two lexical processing routines.

Effects of lip reading on word repetition

A crude characterization of the effects of lip reading in normal subjects is that it can provide additional information about heard speech sounds (see Dodd and Campbell 1987). If MK has a difficulty in phoneme perception, he should then benefit from the opportunity to gain additional information from the speaker's lips. If, on the other hand, as we have argued, MK has no primary difficulty in speech sound analysis, he will not benefit from the additional information about speech sounds that lip reading can provide. We therefore presented him with a list of 200 items for repetition in two separate sessions two weeks apart. On half the items in each session he was encouraged to watch the speaker's face; in the other half her face was concealed.

---

8. We have recently been working with a patient who, although he is worse than MK in phoneme discrimination, can repeat more than 60% of monosyllabic nonwords correctly. We can therefore be confident that MK's phoneme perception is good enough to support some nonword repetition.

The results are straightforward. MK repeated 58/200 words correctly when lip reading was encouraged, and 58/200 when lip reading was prevented. Lip reading clearly has no effect on the accuracy of his word repetition. This provides further support for our claim that a difficulty in speech sound analysis does not underlie his difficulties in auditory word recognition or oral word repetition.

Effects of word imageability on oral repetition and writing to dictation

To assess the effects of imageability on oral repetition and writing to dictation, we used two lists of matched high and low imageability words. The results for the matched sets of high and low frequency words of high and low imageability are presented in table 23. In oral repetition the effect of word frequency is not significant (Fisher exact test, $z = .90$, ns), and the imageability effect only approaches statistical significance ($z = 1.35$, $p < .10$). In writing to dictation, there is a significant effect of imageability ($z = 2.47$, $p < .01$), but there is no significant effect of word frequency ($z = 0.67$, ns).

In the list of 100 high imageability words matched to 100 low imageability words, MK performs very much better with the high imageability items in both oral repetition ($z = 4.40$, $p < .001$) and writing to dictation ($z = 2.93$, $p < .002$).

It is clear that his ability to repeat words aloud and to write them to dictation is affected by the stimulus word's imageability, indicating that

Table 23
The effects of word imageability on oral word repetition and writing to dictation
(i) **List of high and low imageability words of high and low frequency from Howard (1987)**

| | | Proportion correct | | |
| | | Oral | Writing to | |
	N	repetition	dictation	Examples
Low imag., high freq. words	20	.45	.40	IDEA, ANSWER
Low imag., low freq. words	20	.20	.15	SPAN, PARDON
High imag., high freq. words	20	.50	.55	ROAD, DOCTOR
High imag., low freq. words	20	.50	.60	HAWK, INFANT

(ii) **List of high and low imageability words matched exactly for word frequency and letter length**

| | | Proportion correct | | |
| | | Oral | Writing to | |
	N	repetition	dictation	Examples
High imageability words	100	.60	.48	SKIRT, GRASS, BOMB
Low imageability words	100	.29	.26	BLAME, FAULT, SOUL

he must at least sometimes be using a 'semantic routine' to perform both tasks. If he is ever relying on a semantic routine alone, we would expect that semantic errors should occur in both oral repetition and writing to dictation.

Analysis of errors in oral repetition and writing to dictation of high and low imageability words

Table 24 presents an analysis of MK's errors with the 100 high imageability words and 100 low imageability words in oral repetition and writing to dictation.

As predicted, *semantic* errors occur in both tasks. They occur with both high and low imageability stimuli. In both tasks there are, in Coltheart's (1980b) terms, both 'shared feature errors' (e.g., 'stupid' → 'silly'; 'engine' → MACHINE) and 'associate errors' (e.g., 'type' → 'sheet'; 'autumn' → LEAVES).

Phonologically related errors are common in both tasks. Arbitrarily we classify under this heading any response when half the phonemes in the response are present in the stimulus in approximately the same order. Of the phonologically related errors in repetition 23/26 are real words; and 28/29 of these errors are real words in writing to dictation. If phonologically related errors resulted from postlexical errors in output, we would expect only a small proportion of real word errors; and they would be only accidentally real words—in Butterworth's (1979) phrase, 'jargon homophones'. But the proportions of real words are far too high to allow for an explanation of this kind; instead the errors must result from addressing of phonologically similar lexical entries in either input or output. The errors in writing to dictation in most cases resemble the stimulus both phonologically and orthographically. One of the writing errors ('gaol' → GOAL) resembles the stimulus only in orthography, so we have classified this separately as a spelling error. Some of the other errors resemble the stimulus in phonology and not orthography (e.g., 'motion' → OCEAN; 'fear' → SPHERE), so we have some confidence in a source of these errors at a phonological level.

The majority of errors in both tasks bear no obvious relationship to the target. We have subdivided these errors into three categories: *neologisms* are nonwords that bear no relationship to the target, and *perseverations* are real words that bear no relationship to the target but have occurred earlier in the session as either correct responses or errors. Other *unrelated real word* errors are classified as that.

There are a few errors of other types: there is one addition of an inflectional suffix in oral repetition and one inflectional and two derivational errors in writing to dictation. Some errors are ambiguous between the categories of phonologically and semantically related errors (e.g.,

Table 24
Analysis of the responses in oral repetition and writing to dictation of 100 high imageability words and 100 matched low imageability words

(i) **Oral word repetition**

| Response types | No. of responses with | | Examples |
	high imag.	low imag.	
Correct repetition	60	29	
Derivational/inflectional errors	0	1	'rate' → 'rates'
Semantic errors	8	7	'factory' → 'steel'
			'learn' → 'know'
Phonologically related real words	7	16	'missile' → 'whistle'
			'trim' → 'swim'
Unrelated real words	13	25	'shirt' → 'iron'
			'push' → 'pillow'
Phonologically related nonword responses	1	2	'jacket' → '/tʃɑk/'
			'merit' → '/'merə/'
Neologisms (unrelated nonwords)	1	4	'land' → '/'pælaʊ/'
			'patent' → '/'fæntaʊ/'
Perseverations	7	13	'ball' → 'together'
			'dare' → 'together'
Other responses	3	3	

(ii) **Writing to dictation**

| Response types | No. of responses with | | Examples |
	high imag.	low imag.	
Correct written word	48	26	
Derivational/inflectional errors	3	0	'lunch' → LUNCHEON
Semantic errors	10	6	'lady' → GIRL
			'reply' → YES
Phonologically related real words	11	17	'skirt' → SQUIRT
			'origin' → ORANGE
Unrelated real words	20	27	'sheep' → NEEDLE
			'theme' → SLOW
Spelling error	1	0	'goal' → GOAL
Phonologically related nonwords	0	1	'merit' → MERROW
Neologisms (unrelated nonwords)	2	6	'porch' → RUNCH
			'prime' → BRANY
Perseverations	4	6	'ball' → TOGETHER
			'neutral' → TOGETHER
Other responses	1	11	

'penny' → MONEY; 'winter' → WIND; 'prime' → 'prize'). The other errors appear to result from two errors of different types in sequence: for example a phonological and then semantic error ('amount' → REIN [via MOUNT?]), phonological and then morphological errors ('nice' → 'mouse' [via MICE?]; 'mature' → IMPURE [via PURE?]), and spelling errors superimposed on mistakes of various kinds (e.g., 'modest' → QUIETE; 'device' → DEVINE).

There are no examples of omissions or failures to produce a response. MK appears to interpret the task as requiring in all circumstances a response of some kind. Many or all of the perseverations and other apparently unrelated responses may represent responses that he has generated in the absence of any relevant information from the stimulus word.

Semantic errors in repetition and writing to dictation: a chance effect?

In both oral repetition and writing to dictation, MK makes a substantial proportion of errors that are (apparently) unrelated to the target. As Ellis and Marshall (1978) point out, unrelated errors will sometimes by chance bear some semantic resemblance to the target. In this analysis we will try to establish whether MK's semantic errors can be attributed to chance semantic similarity, or whether there is a genuine semantic resemblance between the stimulus words and his responses.

From MK's repetition errors on the two hundred words of the Bauer and Stanovich (1980) list, we took all 68 responses that were not phonologically related to the target. We then randomly reassigned the responses to the stimulus words (with the constraint that stimulus and response could not be the same). For each stimulus word, we then had a genuine error and a pseudo-error generated by random reallocation. These were put into random order in two halves; each stimulus word occurred in the same position in the list in each half once with the genuine error and once with the pseudo-error. These lists of pairs of words were then given to three normal people, who were asked to judge on a 0–3 scale whether the pairs of words were closely associated (3), quite associated (2), distantly associated (1), or unrelated in meaning (0). We then took the median rating of the three judges for each item. If there really are semantic errors in MK's repetition, then more of the genuine errors should be judged to be semantically associated than the pseudo-errors (where the degree of resemblance is due only to chance). The identical procedure was followed with MK's 76 phonologically unrelated errors in writing to dictation on the same lists.

The results are shown in table 25. The genuine errors are judged significantly more closely related than the pseudo-errors both in oral repetition (Wilcoxon test, $z = 3.59$, $p < .001$) and in writing to dictation ($z = 2.74$, $p < .003$). We can therefore be sure that MK really is making some semantically related errors in both oral repetition and writing to dictation, and the

Table 25
Judgments of semantic relatedness of error responses. Three subjects were asked to judge
how closely associated were MK's errors, and pseudo-errors generated by randomly
re-allocating the responses to the stimuli. The results are based on the median of the the
three judges. (Errors are all incorrect responses where the response was phonologically
unrelated to the target on the 200 items in the Bauer and Stanovich (1980) lists)

	Unrelated	Response judged Distantly related	Quite related	Closely related
Errors in oral repetition				
MK's errors	24	17	15	11
pseudo-errors	40	19	7	2
Errors in writing to dictation				
MK's errors	29	21	14	12
pseudo-errors	39	24	10	3

degree of resemblance cannot be accounted for by chance. The degree of
semantic similarity between stimuli and genuine errors is the same in oral
repetition and writing to dictation ($\chi^2(3) = 0.41$; ns).

Spelling errors: a role for phonological-to-orthographic conversion processes?

It is clear that for MK both oral repetition and writing to dictation involve
semantic mediation. Genuine semantic errors occur, performance is affected
by imageability, and his failure with nonwords indicates that he sublexical
routines are unavailable. For oral repetition, within the model we are using
there is a single semantic routine. For writing to dictation there are three
different routines, which differ in the way in which a representation in the
cognitive system accesses output orthography. In figure 4, routine C goes
directly CS → GOL → GOB. Routine D runs CS → POL → GOL → GOB, and as
noted above its signature will be homophone errors superimposed on
semantic errors. Routine E runs from CS → POL → POB → GOB (via subword
level P → O conversion); its signature will be phonologically plausible
nonword spelling errors.

We therefore examined the set of errors in writing to dictation MK made
on a set of 530 words, drawn from a variety of stimulus lists, to see
whether there was any evidence of the error types that would indicate he is
using routines D or E.

There is a single possible example of a homophone error superimposed
on a semantic error: 'paw' written as CLAUSE. We suspect that this error is
not a chance resemblance between stimulus and response, because in word
repetition MK made the identical error repeating 'paw' as '/klɔz/' (i.e.,
claws/clause). Even if MK does use routine D often, he would probably

make few errors, simply because of the small number of words that he produces as semantic errors that have homophones with different spellings. Because the nature of his semantic errors in writing to dictation is beyond our control, we can see no experimental manipulation that we could use to increase the incidence of these errors, which is, we think, the only way to confirm that MK does use a phonologically mediated but lexical routine in writing to dictation.

Evidence for MK's use of sublexical phonologically mediated information in writing to dictation is much easier to collect. If his spelling errors in writing to dictation result from the use of phonological information, then we would expect that the errors will be phonologically plausible. If, on the other hand, they reflect simply a breakdown in spelling, due for example to loss of information about the correct letters, the errors will occur on any letter, whether the result is phonologically plausible or not.

On the set of 530 responses in writing to dictation, he made 38 errors that were nonwords. Of these 10 were clearly target related, and 7 of these are phonologically plausible errors (in MK's accent). Typically these involve misspelling of vowels (as in 'disaster' → DESASTER; 'widow' → WEDOW; and 'hurricane' → HARRICANE), but consonants too are involved (e.g., 'chocolate' → CHOCKOLATE). The other errors involve letter misordering (DIFFODAL; TENGARINE) or addition ('truth' → THRUTH).

Of the other nonword responses 11/28 could have been pronounced as a real word. A few of the responses appear to be due to phonologically based errors superimposed on semantic errors (e.g., 'prime' → BRANY; 'thermometer' → TEMPEATER; 'stupid' → SILLOW). Other responses, while they are apparently phonologically plausible renderings of real words, bear no obvious relationship to the target (e.g., 'saw' → STOAL; 'ball' → DOW; 'step' → DOUT). The remainder of his unrelated nonword responses in writing to dictation could not be pronounced as real words, but they almost always obey the rules that govern permissible sequences of English letters (i.e., they are 'orthotactically legal'; e.g., 'honest' → OWALL, 'river' → DRUPFUL, 'blonde' → HOUGHTER). It is clear, however, that many more of these nonword responses can be pronounced as real words than we would expect by chance. Thus both MK's target related and other nonword responses in writing to dictation betray the fact that phonological information is used to constrain MK's spelling responses. There is, then, clear evidence that at least on some occasions in writing to dictation MK uses routine E, which depends on subword level phonological-to-orthographic conversion.

The effects of part of speech on oral repetition and writing to dictation

We used the same three lists that we had used with oral reading, to assess whether there was for MK a difference between performance with 'content' and 'function' words in oral repetition and writing to dictation. The first list, from Patterson (1979), consists of sets matched for word frequency and letter length, but not for imageability. The second list consists of word sets closely matched for imageability, but only approximately for frequency and length. The final list is matched precisely in terms of frequency and length, but not in terms of imageability. To assess whether there were any differences between nouns and verbs, we used a list provided by Alan Allport, with words matched in terms of imageability, frequency, and length.

The results are shown in table 26. In the Patterson lists there is no significant difference between function and content words in either task; in the imageability matched lists there is a trend toward a difference in oral word repetition, which does not reach significance (Fisher exact, $z = 1.43$; $p = .076$ one-tailed); in writing to dictation, the difference is not significant ($z = 0.76$; $p = 0.22$). In the third list, which is not matched in terms of word imageability, there is a significant advantage for content words in both tasks (oral word repetition, $z = 2.39$, $p < .01$; writing to dictation, $z = 2.58$, $p < .005$). However, as imageability *does* affect MK's performance, this need only reflect an effect of imageability rather than one of part of speech *per se*.

These results, then, do not demonstrate that there is a difference in performance between content and function words, once imageability is controlled. But we should emphasize that, equally, they do not demonstrate that there is *no effect* of part of speech. In the imageability-matched lists, the 95% confidence interval for the difference in proportion of words of each type correct is .28 to $-.01$ in repetition and .24 to $-.07$ in writing to dictation. These results are therefore compatible with a quite substantial advantage for content words over function words. As the word sets used in this list represent all the available words in the MRC database from the overlapping imageability range, this issue cannot be definitively resolved without new matching data.

'Deep dyslexic' patients are said to not only perform worse in reading with function words than content words, but also to produce function word errors to function word stimuli (Marshall and Newcombe 1966). In order to assess whether this applied to MK's oral word repetition and writing to dictation, we analyzed his errors on the imageability matched lists. In repetition, there are function word responses to both content word stimuli (e.g., 'entire' → 'together') and function word stimuli ('above' → 'enough'). Function word responses make up 15 of the 32 real word errors to function word stimuli, and only 8 of the 36 real word errors to content word stimuli; this difference is significant (Fisher exact, $z = 1.87$; $p = .03$, one-tailed). In writing to dictation of these lists, there is a similar pattern.

Table 26
The effects of word class in oral word repetition and writing to dictation

(i) List of 'content' and 'function' words from Patterson (1979)

		Proportion correct	
	N	Oral repetition	Writing to dictation
'Function words'	60	.13	.05
'Content words'	60	.20	.08

(ii) List of 'content' and 'function' words matched approximately for imageability (for details see text)

		Proportion correct		
	N	Oral repetition	Writing to dictation	Examples
'Function words'	40	.10	.20	BOTH, OVER
'Content words'	60	.23	.23	KEEP, REASON

(iii) List of 'content' and 'function' words matched exactly for word frequency and letter length

		Proportion correct		
	N	Oral repetition	Writing dictation	Examples
'Function words'	50	.10	.04	DID, US, EVER
'Content words'	50	.30	.24	MAN, GO, NEED

(iv) Lists of matched nouns and verbs, from Allport and Funnell (1981)

		Proportion correct		
	N	Oral repetition	Writing to dictation	Examples
Nouns	30	.30	.20	FAITH, FUND
Verbs	30	.37	.20	SERVE, WEAR

Function word responses occur both with content word stimuli (e.g., 'keep' → AGAIN) and function word stimuli ('had' → WAS). But with content word stimuli there are 6 function word errors in 42 real word errors, while with function word stimuli there are 15 function word responses in 29 real word errors; this difference is significant ($z = 3.11; p < .001$). Thus, in both word repetition and writing to dictation, function word error responses occur most often with function word stimuli, even in imageability matched lists with mixed presentation. Even though there is no significant difference between the word classes in terms of accuracy, there is a difference in the types of errors that they elicit.

The results of the comparison between nouns and verbs in oral word repetition and writing to dictation are shown in table 26. There are no differences between nouns and verbs in either task.

The effects of word syllable length on oral repetition and writing to dictation

Patients with problems in the phonological organization of spoken output may have greater difficulty in producing longer rather than shorter words. McCarthy and Warrington (1984), for example, report a patient who made phonological errors in oral repetition, oral word reading, and spontaneous speech who performed particularly poorly in repetition of longer words (see Caplan, Vanier, and Baker 1986; Pate, Saffran, and Schwartz 1987).

On the other hand, a patient who has lost some information in an input lexicon would be expected to perform worse with short words than with longer ones. This is because short words have more neighbors that differ by only one phoneme or feature—it is easy to mistake 'cat' for 'pat', 'cap', 'cot', etc., whereas 'crocodile' cannot easily be misidentified as another word. We have already presented a number of lines of evidence that MK has lost some of the distinctiveness between entries in a phonological input lexicon: he is relatively poor at auditory lexical decision, compared with his performance with the same words presented visually; he misdefines words as phonologically-similar real words (e.g., 'cult' → 'a horse' [COLT]); he makes phonologically related real word errors in both oral repetition and writing to dictation. In auditory comprehension we showed that MK's performance was worse with short words than long words. Since we have argued that in both oral word repetition and writing to dictation MK relies on a semantic routine, he should show better performance with longer words in both tasks.

He was presented with a mixed list made up of thirty mono-, thirty bi-, and thirty trisyllabic words matched for imageability and frequency (for matching data see appendix 1). In separate sessions he read them aloud, repeated them, and wrote them to dictation.

Table 27
The effects of word syllable length on oral word repetition, writing to dictation, and oral word reading

	N	Proportion correct Oral repetition	Writing to dictation	Oral reading
One-syllable words	30	.73	.73	.97
Two-syllable words	30	.63	.77	.80
Three-syllable words	30	.90	.70	.73
Total		.76	.73	.83

The results are shown in table 27. In oral word repetition there is a significant advantage for longer words (Jonckheere trend test, $z = 1.64$, $p = .05$), but in writing to dictation there is no effect ($z = -.15$; ns). In oral reading, by contrast, and in accordance with the reading results reported earlier, MK is better with the *shorter* words ($z = 2.24$; $p < .05$).

The error patterns show why we failed to find the predicted advantage for longer words in writing to dictation. Spelling errors (that is nonword responses that are orthographically related to the target) do not occur with one-syllable words, twice with two-syllable words (CHOCKOLATE; 'widow' → WEDOW), and seven times with three-syllable words (e.g., HARRICANE; CROCADALE; DIFFODAL). We have already shown that errors of this kind must represent failures in output when the appropriate orthographic output lexicon entry had been accessed. This confirms our findings in the analysis of influences on written picture naming; there too MK showed a significant tendency to make errors with longer stimuli. If, to compensate for this, we count correct responses and spelling errors, there is a significant length effect in writing to dictation (Jonckheere trend test, $z = 2.26$, $p < .05$). MK therefore has superior ability to spell shorter words, which cancels out the effects in writing to dictation of his superior ability to recognize longer words.

The effects of inflectional and derivational suffixes on oral repetition and writing to dictation

Patients who have previously been reported to make semantic errors in repetition, or in writing to dictation, have usually also made morphological errors, by adding, deleting, or substituting derivational or inflectional affixes (e.g., Michel 1979; Bub and Kertesz 1982). In the error analysis presented above there were very few errors of this kind, but all the stimuli involved were single morphemes; the rarity of morphological errors may simply reflect the fact that affix addition errors are relatively uncommon.

We therefore presented MK with a set of words that were derived from 75 morphologically simple roots. Each of these roots occurred once as the root, once with an inflectional suffix (*-ing, -(e)s,* and *-ed* each occurred 25 times), and once with a derivational suffix (*-y, -ist, -ly, -ful,* and *-age* each occurred 15 times). Thus we had, for example:

Root	Inflected form	Derived form
DRAIN	DRAINING	DRAINAGE
NOVEL	NOVELS	NOVELIST
CLEAN	CLEANING	CLEANLY
JUMP	JUMPED	JUMPY
HOPE	HOPING	HOPEFUL

The words were assigned to three lists so that each stem occurred only once in each list, and there were equal proportions of roots, inflected, and derived forms in each list. These lists were presented for oral repetition, writing to dictation and oral reading.

The results are shown in table 28. In reading there is a significant advantage for roots over the two suffixed forms (Cochran $Q(2) = 7.11$; $p < .05$); nearly all the errors are, as in other reading tasks, 'phonologically plausible'. The difference between the conditions simply reflects the advan-

Table 28
The effects of derivational and inflectional suffixes on MK's performance in oral repetition, writing to dictation, and oral word reading ($n = 75$ for words of each type)

(i) **Oral word repetition**

	Proportion correct	Proportion suffix error	Proportion other error
Root form	.56	.07	.37
Inflected form	.15	.51	.35
Derived form	.41	.29	.29

(ii) **Writing to dictation**

	Proportion correct	Proportion suffix error	Proportion other error
Root form	.56	.09	.35
Inflected form	.05	.59	.36
Derived form	.32	.33	.35

(iii) **Oral word reading**

	Proportion correct	Proportion suffix error	Proportion other error
Root form	.95	.03	.03
Inflected form	.84	.05	.11
Derived form	.84	.03	.13

tage in MK's reading for shorter words, which we have already documented. The infrequency of suffix errors and the equal performance on the two suffixed sets that are of equal length supports this view.

In oral word repetition there is a significant difference between the three conditions ($Q(2) = 27.96$; $p < .001$), and the root is repeated significantly better than the derived form, and the derived form significantly better than the inflected form. The greater difficulty with inflected than derived forms is accounted for by a higher rate of suffix errors; with both inflections and derivations the majority of suffix errors are deletions (71% of suffix errors in each case). The remaining suffix errors are substitutions.

The pattern of results in writing to dictation is, in effect, identical: there is a significant difference between the three conditions ($Q(2) = 40.91$; $p < .001$), and the root is written significantly better than the derived form, and the derived form significantly better than the inflected form. The greater difficulty with inflected than with derived forms is completely accounted for by a higher rate of suffix errors; with both inflections and derivations the majority of suffix errors are deletions (80% of suffix errors with inflections, and 93% with derivations).

Both the derived and inflected forms are very close to the root in both meaning and phonological form; errors reflecting phonological and/or semantic similarity between root and suffixed forms should therefore distribute approximately equally between inflected and derived forms. That MK is so very much poorer with inflected than derived forms demonstrates that there is a specific difficulty with words with inflectional suffixes. It is clear therefore that genuine morphological errors do occur in MK's oral word repetition and writing to dictation, when he is presented with suffixed words.

The effects of spelling regularity on oral repetition and writing to dictation

In oral picture naming, MK sometimes made orthographically based errors. We argued that these errors occurred when MK failed to access the correct entry in the phonological output lexicon but did manage to access the appropriate entry in the graphemic output lexicon. He then converted this output orthographic code into an input code which he read via the sublexical reading routine, thus generating an orthographically based error in oral naming.

We have argued that when MK repeats spoken words he uses the 'semantic routine'. The output part of this process is identical to the output process involved in oral picture naming; accordingly, we should predict that orthographically based errors may occur in the oral repetition of irregularly spelled words, just as they do in naming. We therefore presented him with the Bauer and Stanovich (1980) list of 100 regular and 100

Table 29
The effects of spelling regularity on oral word repetition and writing to dictation; word sets from Bauer and Stanovich (1980)

| | N | Proportion correct | |
		Oral repetition	Writing to dictation
Regular words	100	.29	.36
Irregular words	100	.35	.40

irregular words for oral repetition[9]. As can be seen from table 29, there is no overall effect of spelling regularity on MK's accuracy in repetition. Only two errors have an apparent orthographic source: 'move' → 'mauve', and 'gross' → 'cross' (which if orthographically based involved a phonological error as well). In all the repetition data we find only three other examples of errors that convincingly incorporate an orthographic element:

'move'   → '/məʊv/'
'palm'   → '/pælmə/'
'mortgage' → '/mɔtgeɪʤ/'

This evidence suggests that MK occasionally uses orthographic information in oral word repetition, but certainly not as often as he does in oral picture naming.

The data in table 29 on the effect of word regularity on writing to dictation confirm again our claim that MK does not use a sub-lexical routine in this task. Instead he uses a 'semantic' routine, on which spelling regularity has no effect.

Analysis of errors in oral repetition and writing to dictation

In order to investigate further the factors causing errors of different types, we assembled the results from oral repetition and writing to dictation for 440 morphologically simple content words gathered from a number of different lists. From these we selected the words that had imageability values in the MRC Psycholinguistic Database. These values, which can vary from 100–700, are derived from judgments on a seven-point scale; the higher the value the more 'imageable' the item is judged to be. Where a word in this set had been presented in more than one list, we selected one of the responses at random. This yielded a final set of 367 words together

---

9. Words that are 'regular' for reading are not necessarily 'regular' for spelling. This does not concern us too much: as Hatfield and Patterson (1983) point out, the words that have 'irregular' spelling-to-sound correspondences are likely to have more exceptional sound-to-spelling correspondences than the 'regular' words.

Table 30
The characteristics of words giving rise to responses of different types in oral word repetition

Response type	N	Imageability			Log word frequency.			Word length		
		Mean	s.d.	s.e.	Mean	s.d.	s.e.	Mean	s.d.	s.e.
Correct	146	532	103	8	1.60	.48	.04	4.14	1.88	.10
Inflectional/derivational error	6	466	118	48	1.51	.66	.27	3.83	1.17	.48
Semantic error	27	508	119	23	1.53	.69	.13	3.96	1.22	.24
Phonologically related real word	52	462	114	16	1.52	.48	.07	3.83	.92	.13
Phonological/ semantic error	3	465	105	61	1.41	.40	.23	3.67	.58	.33
Nonword responses	25	492	107	22	1.61	.55	.11	4.04	1.31	.26
Unrelated real words (inc. perseverations)	103	478	115	11	1.55	.42	.04	3.67	1.00	.10
Complex errors	5	404	117	52	1.61	.50	.22	3.2	.84	.37

with the responses that they had elicited in oral repetition and writing to dictation.

We examined the effects of three different factors: stimulus word imageability, log-transformed Kucera and Francis word frequency, and word length in phonemes. Over the set of 367 items none of these factors were significantly correlated with each other (imageability × frequency, $r = -0.17$; imageability × length, $r = -0.12$; frequency × length, $r = -0.05$). We can therefore assume that the effects of these three variables will not be confounded.

The characteristics of the words giving rise to responses of different kinds in oral repetition are given in table 30. Words that give rise to correct responses are significantly higher in imageability than words that give rise to errors (mean imageability correct 538, errors 478; $t(365) = 4.59$, $p < .001$), and significantly longer (mean phoneme length correct 4.15, errors 3.78, $t(365) = 3.11$, $p < .01$), but there is no difference in log word frequency (mean log frequency correct 1.60, errors 1.55, $t(365) = 1.04$, ns). Words that give rise to phonologically related real word errors are significantly lower in imageability ($t(196) = 4.07$, $p < .001$) and significantly shorter than the words that are repeated correctly ($t(196) = 1.78$, $p < .05$). Words that give rise to unrelated real word errors are also both lower in imageability ($t(247) = 3.88$, $p < .001$) and shorter than words that yield correct responses ($t(247) = 3.34$, $p < .001$). On the other hand, words that give rise to semantic errors do not differ significantly from those that are correctly repeated in imageability, frequency, or length.

Table 31
The characteristics of words giving rise to responses of different types in writing to dictation

Response type	N	Imageability			Log word frequency			Word length		
		Mean	s.d.	s.e.	Mean	s.d.	s.e.	Mean	s.d.	s.e.
Correct	143	533	101	8	1.58	.47	.04	4.02	1.12	.09
Inflectional/derivational error	10	500	124	39	1.45	.44	.14	3.60	.97	.31
Semantic error	36	531	95	16	1.55	.67	.11	3.63	1.22	.20
Phonologically related real word	48	470	122	17	1.51	.49	.07	3.92	.90	.13
Phonological/ semantic error	4	475	139	69	1.88	.36	.18	3.50	1.29	.64
Nonword responses	16	468	123	31	1.64	.52	.13	3.88	.89	.22
Unrelated real word (inc. perseverations)	95	470	112	12	1.58	.46	.05	3.84	1.11	.11
Complex errors	15	406	103	27	1.54	.37	.10	4.67	1.54	.40

In repetition, then, correct responses and semantic errors are found particularly with words that are both higher in imageability, and longer. Phonologically related real word and unrelated real word errors are found most frequently with words that are lower in imageability or shorter. This confirms a number of results in the experiments described above: repetition is better for high imageability words than for low imageability words; repetition is better for longer words than for shorter ones; phonological confusions in lexical decision and repetition seem to occur most frequently with abstract words.

In writing to dictation, the identical pattern of results is found as in repetition for the effects of word imageability, but there are no significant effects of either log transformed word frequency or word phoneme length (table 31). Words that are written correctly are significantly higher in imageability than those that result in errors (mean imageability correct 533, errors 477, $t(365) = 4.78$, $p < .001$). Words that result in phonologically related real word errors are significantly lower in imageability than those that result in correct writing ($t(189) = 3.57$, $p < .001$) and less imageable than those that elicit semantic errors ($t(82) = 2.49$, $p < .02$). Words that elicit unrelated real word errors are also significantly lower in imageability than those that result in correct writing ($t(237) = 4.46$, $p < .001$) and less imageable than those that elicit semantic errors ($t(130) = 2.83$, $p < .01$). Our failure to find a word length effect in writing to dictation is attributable to the output spelling difficulty, which offsets the advantage for longer words in auditory lexical access.

The relative imageability and frequency of stimuli and error responses

MK makes phonologically related real word errors in both word repetition and writing to dictation. The analogous errors in oral reading are errors that are visually related to the stimulus. For a patient (KF) who made semantic errors in oral reading of single words (a 'deep dyslexic'), Shallice and Warrington (1975) demonstrated that his visual reading errors were on average significantly more concrete than the stimuli that produced them.

To investigate whether there is any systematic relationship between the word frequency and imageability of MK's error responses of different kinds and the errors that elicited them, we conducted two further analyses. We were interested in the three commonest error types: semantic errors, phonologically related errors, and unrelated responses in oral repetition and writing to dictation. Comparisons of imageability were done by asking normal subjects to judge the relative imageability of stimuli and responses. Frequency was assessed by comparison of Kucera and Francis frequencies.

The results were uniformly negative, and so will not be reported in any detail; the full results are available from the authors on request. There was no evidence that responses of any kind in either task differed systematically in imageability from the words that elicited them; and there was no evidence that words produced as errors of these kinds were of higher frequency than the words that elicited them.

A comparison of MK's performance in spoken and written naming of 100 pictures and oral repetition and writing to dictation of their names

In all the comparisons between oral repetition and writing to dictation that we have reported, there is a marked degree of similarity between MK's performance in the two tasks. Overall error rates are very similar; patterns of errors are very similar; the same variables, in general, affect performance in each task. We have argued that this similarity reflects a breakdown in the processing routines that these two tasks have in common—recognition of a heard word in the auditory input lexicon, and access on the basis of this to central semantic representations. In discussing MK's performance in picture naming, we argued that output of both spoken and written names on the basis of central semantic representations was only mildly impaired; but again we argued that there was quantitative and qualitative similarity between spoken and written naming. We should therefore predict that oral repetition and writing to dictation will be severely impaired relative to spoken and written picture naming, because repetition and writing to dictation both involve the additional use of MK's impaired auditory input processes. We argued that phonologically related real word errors result from misrecognition at the level of the auditory input lexicon; these errors

Table 32
A comparison of word repetition, writing to dictation, oral and written naming of a set of
100 picture names

	Word repetition	Writing to dictation	Spoken naming	Written naming
Correct responses	39	47	82	77
Errors				
Inflectional errors	3	1	1	—
Semantic errors	7	8	14	19
Phonologically related real words	15	13	1	—
Unrelated real words	26	23	—	—
Nonword responses	10	5	1	4
Others	—	3	1	—

should therefore be found exclusively in oral repetition and writing to dictation. In discussing MK's naming performance, we argued that semantic errors with picturable words arose in the process of output from the semantic system. We would therefore predict that semantic errors should be found in oral repetition, writing to dictation, and spoken and written naming.

Table 32 presents the comparison between oral repetition, writing to dictation, and spoken and written picture naming for the pictures of the '100 item' naming test. Consistent with the previous results, performance in oral repetition and writing to dictation are very similar in accuracy and variety of errors. Spoken and written naming are also very similar but very much better than oral repetition and writing to dictation. Phonologically related real word errors occur almost exclusively in oral repetition and writing to dictation, which supports our claim that they reflect a breakdown in auditory input processes. Semantic errors, however, occur in all four tasks, and in each task they are in a similar ratio to correct responses; with concrete, picturable items, semantic errors probably reflect a breakdown in output once the appropriate semantic representation has been accessed.

Summary of MK's performance in oral repetition and writing to dictation

Overall accuracy is very similar in oral repetition and writing to dictation. The same variables affect performance in the two tasks: in oral repetition and writing to dictation MK's performance is better with high imageability words than low imageability words, better with morphologically simple words than with affixed words, better with words with derivational suffixes than words with inflectional suffixes. In both oral repetition and writing to dictation there is no effect of part of speech in lists where imageability is closely controlled, no effect of word frequency, and no effect oᶜ spelling regularity. Only in the effects of word length is there a dissociation; whereas MK's repetition performance is more accurate with longer words than shorter ones, in writing to dictation there is no length effect. This, we demonstrated, was due to (output) spelling errors, which tend to occur more often with longer words, counteracting the effect of MK's better input for longer words than for shorter ones.

The same error types occur in both tasks: morphological errors, semantic errors, phonologically related real word errors, and unrelated errors. In both tasks function word errors are found most frequently with function word stimuli. Semantic errors and correct responses occur particularly with high imageability word stimuli; phonologically related real word errors and unrelated real word errors occur particularly with low imageability stimuli. There is no overall tendency for error responses of any type to be more or less imageable or more frequent than the responses that elicit them.

The data from naming tasks that we presented earlier show that, at least with picturable items, MK's written and spoken output from the semantic system is, at most, mildly impaired. His difficulties in oral word repetition and writing to dictation are, by comparison, severe. Because (i) MK makes semantic errors, and (ii) performance is affected by a semantic factor (imageability), we have argued that he relies on a semantic routine for both oral word repetition and writing to dictation. It seems most likely that impairment in both tasks reflects a common impairment in access to central semantic representations from auditory input. The properties of MK's impairment in auditory word comprehension should therefore correspond to the properties of his impairment in oral word repetition and writing to dictation.

As we showed in our discussion of MK's comprehension, his auditory input processes, like oral word repetition and writing to dictation, are better for high imageability words than low imageability words, and like his word repetition performance, auditory comprehension is better for long words than short words. In auditory comprehension, in oral word repetition, and in writing to dictation, MK sometimes makes errors reflecting access to partial semantic information from the stimulus, and sometimes makes errors reflecting misidentification of the word as another, phonologically similar item. We claim, therefore, that there is an impairment in auditory comprehension processes that is reflected not only in the characteristics of his impairment in auditory comprehension but also in oral word repetition and writing to dictation, both of which rely on a semantic routine.

Chapter 10
Delayed Copying

We have so far reported on MK's performance in three tasks involving lexical input and lexical output—oral word reading, oral word repetition (spoken responses to written and spoken stimuli, respectively), and writing to dictation (a written response to a spoken stimulus)—but not on producing a written response to a written stimulus.

Copying is often tested by asking the patient to copy a word that remains in full view throughout. This, in relation to lexical processing, is uninteresting; normal people can reproduce words in scripts that are entirely unknown to them by copying stroke-by-stroke. The relevant task for our investigations is delayed copying: the patient is shown a word, which is then removed; only then can the patient produce a written response. In this sense delayed copying is the direct analogue of oral word repetition; the stimulus and response are successive and not simultaneous events.

The lexical model of figure 1 again provides three routines that might be used for copying. We added a 'subword level orthographic-to-graphemic conversion' system, which is not represented in Patterson's (1986) version of the model. This system is needed to account for normal people's ability to copy nonwords; that this is not simply stroke-by-stroke copying is demonstrated by the normal ability to transcribe nonwords from, for example, upper to lower case. There are, it is suggested, two lexical routines available: one is semantically mediated and the other depends on a hypothesized 'direct route' connecting the orthographic input lexicon and the graphemic output lexicon.

To conduct a brief screening of MK's copying abilities, he was tested with a set of words consisting of 10 nonwords, 10 abstract words, 10 irregular words, 10 low frequency words, and 10 function words; they were presented in random order. Each word was exposed for 2 seconds, and there was then a five-second (unfilled) delay before MK was asked to respond. The results (table 33) show that MK made only four errors: two with nonwords (TOOP → LOOP; TULT → TULF) and two with low imageability words (METHOD → MOULD, BOTHER → BROTHER). Overall MK's performance is good. Some errors with nonwords are probably characteristic of any 69-year-old; his sublexical copying routine appears largely undisturbed. With

Table 33
Delayed copying. MK's performance in copying words of various kinds presented for
2 seconds followed by a five-second unfilled delay

Word type	N	Proportion correct	Examples
Nonwords	10	.8	THORK, SLAD
Low imageability words	10	.8	RATE, WISH
Irregular words	10	1.0	BUSY, MOULDY
'Function' words	10	1.0	WERE, EITHER
Low frequency words	10	1.0	WAIF, CANINE
Total	50	.92	

real words MK makes very few errors: it is likely therefore that he has lexical information to supplement his sublexical routine. That his only errors occurred with low imageability words suggests that the semantically mediated routine might be involved; however, where the 'sublexical' routine is working well, it is not easy to establish the characteristics of any lexical routines available.

To examine more closely for effects of imageability, we asked MK to copy the 80 words from the imageability and frequency matched sets; they were presented on a card in lower case, and MK after examining the word had to copy them onto the other side in upper case script. With the first forty items copying was immediate, and in the second half there was a five-second unfilled delay before he was allowed to respond. Overall he made only one error, which was to a low frequency high imageability item (INFANT, copied as UNFONT) in the delayed response condition.

We argued earlier that MK makes output spelling errors that occur preferentially with longer words, in both written naming and writing to dictation. The model in figure 1 requires that the same kinds of errors should occur in delayed copying. To test this, MK was asked to copy a set of eighty words, made up of equal numbers of words of 3, 5, 7, and 9 letters, precisely matched for Kucera and Francis word frequency and word imageability. Words were written on one side of the card in upper case and MK had to copy them onto the other side in lower case. Overall MK made six errors; four with nine-letter words (eg CROCODILE → CROCIDILE, ORCHESTRA → ORCHASTRA) and two with seven-letter words (LOBSTER → LUBSTER, ALCOHOL → ALCOHAL). The effect of word length is significant (Jonckheere trend test, $z = 2.45$, $p < .01$).

It is clear that with MK delayed copying is relatively well preserved; the only clear evidence of impairment is due to spelling errors with longer words, which we had already observed in written naming and writing to dictation.

II
Interpretations and Implications

Chapter 11
Model-Based Interpretation of MK's Problems

This case description provides the first reasonably comprehensive account of single word processing deficits by a patient who makes semantic errors in repetition. His difficulties, however, are not confined to oral repetition; he shows significant impairments in oral word reading, writing to dictation, spoken and written word comprehension, and spoken and written naming. The only word processing 'modality' in which his performance is reasonably intact is delayed copying, and here our testing was not extensive enough to pick up particularly mild or subtle deficits.

From this perspective, one might simply say that MK has a global impairment in word processing common to all modalities and tasks. We have shown, however, that although he has deficits in all these different tasks, the impairments are of very different kinds; thus his performance is affected by different variables, and different types of errors occur. We summarize our results on the effects of different variables on performance modalities in table 34, and the occurrence of different error types in table 35.

In this chapter we will try to demonstrate how this set of results can be attributed to a small number of information processing impairments. Our interpretation will be in terms of our revision of Morton and Patterson's (1980) model of lexical processing. As we said in the introduction, we are using this model primarily because it is the only lexical model that specifies all the word processing routines we have investigated with MK in sufficient detail to permit a discussion of this kind. In the next chapter we will turn to the implications that MK's performance patterns have for lexical theories. We will first summarize the specific impairments we believe to underlie MK's deficits in word processing.

Impairment in the auditory input lexicon

We have shown that MK misidentifies auditorily presented words as other phonologically related words in a number of tasks:

— In judging the correct names for pictures, he accepts 40% of real words and 40% of nonwords that differ from the correct name by a single phoneme.

Table 34
Summary of the effects of variables in various tasks for MK

	Written word comprehension	Oral word reading	Spoken word comprehension	Oral word repetition	Writing to dictation	Spoken naming	Written naming	Auditory lexical decision	Visual lexical decision
Spelling regularity	No effect	Regular > irregular	—	No effect	No effect	—	—	—	No effect
Word length	No effect	Short > long	Long > short	Long > short	No effect	No effect	Short > long	—	—
Word imageability	High > low	High > low	High ≫ low	High ≫ low	High ≫ low	No effect*	No effect*	High > low	Within normal range
Word frequency	No effect	High > low	No effect	No effect	No effect	No effect	No effect	No effect	Very small effect
Presence of a suffix	—	No effect +	—	Root > suffixed	Root > suffixed	—	—	—	—
'Content' v 'function' words	—	No effect	—	No effect +	No effect +	—	—	—	—
Nouns v verbs	—	No effect	—	No effect	No effect	—	—	—	—
Performance with nonwords	Poor with pseudo-homophones	Good	?	Nil	Nil	?	?	Rate of misses = FP rate	Rate of misses = FP rate

— No data available, because it was not tested, or it is impossible to test.

+ There was an effect of this variable, but we were able to show that it was due to a confounding with another variable.

* Result based on a restricted range of the variable, or on a restricted set of stimuli, and therefore to be treated with caution.

~ Variable irrelevant to this task.

Table 35
Error types in different tasks by MK

	Written word comprehension	Oral word reading	Spoken word comprehension	Oral word repetition	Writing to dictation	Spoken naming	Written naming
'Phonologically plausible' errors	No homophone errors	Present	~	Very rare orthographically based errors	Some spelling errors are phonologically plausible	Rare orthographically based errors	None
Semantic errors	Present	None	Present	Present	Present	Present	Present
Phonologically related words	None	Very rare	Present	Present	Present	Rare	Rare
Suffix errors	—	Rare	—	Present	Present	Rare*	Rare*
Unrelated errors	—	None	Rare*	Present	Present	Very rare	Very rare

—No data available, because it was not tested, or it is impossible to test.
~ Error type irrelevant to this task.
*Result based on a restricted set of stimuli, and therefore to be treated with caution.

— In definition of auditorily presented words, he often gives definitions of other similar sounding words (e.g., 'cult' defined as 'a horse'
[cf. COLT]).

— In oral word repetition, and in writing words to spoken dictation,
he often substitutes another, similar sounding real word (e.g., 'trim' →
'swim'; 'motion' → OCEAN). We argued that these errors reflected input phonological errors, because phonologically related real word
errors were very rare in spoken or written naming.

Two further lines of evidence support the hypothesis that MK has an
input lexicon problem. First, we were able to demonstrate that his performance was poor in auditory lexical decision; because he was very much
better at lexical decision with the same words in written form, we can be
confident that this is not because he never knew some of the words.
Second, we predicted that comprehension of longer words should be better
than that of short words, because short words have many close phonological neighbors. Testing this hypothesis using matched sets of words of 1, 2,
and 3 syllables, we were able to show that auditory definition and oral
repetition were better for long words than short words.

This difficulty in identification of heard words cannot be attributable to
any peripheral problem in auditory processing. There are several converging lines of evidence for this:

— His hearing is within normal limits.
— MK's performance on minimal pair tasks and auditory rhyme judgments is not impaired.
— In the name judgment task misidentification of phonologically
similar words (and nonwords) is unrelated to the phonetic similarity
between the foil and the target.
— In repetition, lip reading (which provides additional information
about the identity of the heard word) has no effect on MK's performance.

Furthermore, his performance in short term memory tasks, which we anal-
yse in detail elsewhere (Howard and Franklin 1989), supports this view. For
example, MK can match strings of three auditorily presented nonwords; this
level of performance would seem incompatible with any global problem in
word sound identification. In contrast to MK, other patients who have been
reported to have deficits in word sound identification (such as JS reported
by Caramazza, Berndt, and Basili 1983) show poor performance in minimal
pair judgments, poor auditory rhyme judgments, and severely limited short
term memory for auditorily presented lists. It is clear that MK's primary
problem does not lie in word sound identification but rather in the process
of identification of auditorily presented words.

On the other hand, MK's difficulty in auditory word identification is not independent of the words' semantic properties. In auditory lexical decision he is particularly likely to miss low imageability words, and in oral repetition and writing to dictation phonologically related real word errors occur with words that are significantly more abstract than the correctly identified words. We will return to the relationship between auditory word recognition and semantics in chapter 17.

A central semantic problem, more marked for abstract than concrete items?

In all tasks requiring access to a central semantic representation from verbal input, MK shows a marked superiority for words with high imageability ratings as compared to words with low imageability ratings.[10] This difficulty is evident in the following tasks:

— Definition of abstract words is worse than definition of concrete words with both written and spoken word presentation.
— In comprehension tasks not requiring a spoken response (Coltheart's synonym matching and Shallice's word-to-picture matching), there is an advantage for concrete words over abstract words with both spoken and written word presentation.
— In oral word repetition and writing to dictation he performs better with concrete words than abstract words; we have argued that both of these tasks often involve access to central semantic representations as an intermediate stage (these arguments are summarized below).

While MK performs consistently worse in word comprehension tasks with auditory word presentation than with visual word presentation, the relative advantage for concrete words over abstract words is approximately the same with both modalities of presentation. This strongly suggests that there is both a common, central semantic problem that affects comprehension, particularly comprehension of abstract items, independent of the mode of presentation, as well as a word recognition problem that is specific to spoken input.

For MK there is clearly an imageability affect on tasks requiring semantic access, which occurs independently of the input modality. If he has a central lexical semantic impairment, the same problem with abstract words should be found in output tasks. We have not found a practicable way to

10. We have not tried to establish whether this effect is attributable to differences in the 'high imageability'-'low imageability' dimension, or the 'abstract'-'concrete' dimension. The two ratings are highly correlated, and they are certainly confounded in all the lists we have used. We therefore treat the pairs of terms 'high imageability' and 'concrete', and 'low imageability' and 'abstract' as synonymous.

test directly whether MK has a word retrieval disturbance for abstract items. We have only three sources of evidence on this, and all are weak.

First, in naming with the 100 picture test we were unable to show that name imageability affected naming. By their nature, pictures are restricted to imageable items, so only a very limited range of imageability values was represented. However, with other patients, it is possible to show imageability effects in naming, even within this limited imageability range (Howard 1985a). Second, we pointed out that MK produced appropriately a wide range of abstract words in word definition tasks. Third, the fact that overall his repetition errors show no tendency to be rated as more concrete than the words that elicited them suggests that he has no marked difficulty in producing abstract words.

However, semantic access is not perfect even for concrete words. In the picture name judgment task, MK accepts a substantial number of close semantic distractors with both spoken and written word presentation. On the other hand, he almost always accepts the correct name. This shows that on the basis of a spoken or written word he is able to retrieve a semantic representation that is *underspecified*: it is compatible with both the appropriate picture, and a small set of semantically related items (for further discussion see Butterworth et al. 1984; Howard and Orchard-Lisle 1984).[11]

MK has a semantic level word comprehension problem that is more marked with abstract words than concrete words, but even with concrete words he fails to access a fully specified semantic description. The same difficulty, with abstract words, is not obviously present in spoken output, but it is impossible to show this definitively. The evidence therefore suggests that MK's problems in word comprehension are more likely to be due to a failure in semantic access (from spoken and written word input) rather than to a central storage problem. In naming, MK performs at a level close to normal; in written naming of the items from the 100 picture naming test he made 19 semantic errors. In the name judgment task he accepted 19% of semantically related distractors, when the names were presented in written form. This suggests that for 19% of items MK uses a semantic specification that is underspecified, so that semantic errors can occur in production or in comprehension. On these grounds, we might suspect that MK has a central semantic problem for concrete, picturable items that is responsible for his errors in production and comprehension.

His pattern of performance in the 'Pyramids and Palm Trees' test does not

11. In word-to-picture matching tasks (e.g., Bishop and Byng's LUVS; Kay's test), semantic comprehension errors are comparatively rare; we think this reflects the fact that the distractors in these tasks are not so closely related to the target as in the name judgment task and that the presence of a picture choice serves to direct the patients' attention to the relevant aspects of the word's meaning.

support this view. Making semantic judgments on the picture triads MK makes no errors; yet in naming the pictures he misnames a substantial proportion. His level of performance in the judgments shows that MK does not have a general conceptual/semantic impairment. Two possible explanations could be entertained. The first is that, as Warrington (1975), Beauvois (1982), and Saffran (1982) have suggested, there are separable conceptual and lexical semantic systems; MK's problem would then lie in a deficit to the lexical semantic system leaving the conceptual system intact. The second explanation is that MK's semantic problems in word production and comprehension lie not within a semantic system but in impairments to the processes of access to and output from the semantic system. If there are qualitative differences between word comprehension and production, it will favor the second view. Our evidence that imageability is a powerful determinant of word comprehension, yet has no apparent effect on word production, provides some support for the view that MK's problem lies in access and output. In the next chapter we will return to this in greater detail.

Routines available for word repetition

We showed that MK's word repetition involves semantic mediation on at least some occasions; the evidence for this is the occurrence of semantic errors and an imageability effect in repetition.

   The sublexical routine for repetition is not accessible; in nonword repetition his only responses closely related to the target are real words, even though he knows that he is being presented with nonwords. This suggests that he can only use a lexical routine, even in attempting to repeat nonwords. His difficulty with nonwords is not due to any difficulty in nonword production; MK can read short nonwords with quite reasonable levels of accuracy—clearly he can assemble and articulate nonwords. Nor is his difficulty in nonword repetition due to impaired analysis of the auditory nonword input; he can perform minimal pair judgments on nonwords with quite reasonable accuracy. Thus, by elimination, his difficulty in nonword repetition lies in the process of 'subword level auditory-to-phonological conversion'.

   Whether MK has a direct lexical repetition route available is less easy to establish. If we assume, following Morton (1979), that in normal people there is a direct mapping from each unit in the auditory input lexicon to the corresponding entry in the phonological output lexicon, then, where this mapping is intact, patients will be able to repeat any familiar (i.e., lexically represented) word. Because MK's real word repetition is severely impaired, a direct route of this kind cannot be intact. Whether it is impaired or entirely unavailable is less clear. The trouble is that we have no characterization of an impaired direct route. By analogy with the 'direct route' for reading words aloud, we might follow Bub et al. (1985) in suggesting that a defective direct route would work more effectively for high frequency than for low frequency words. If this is true, MK has no 'direct route' for word repetition; word frequency does not affect his repetition.

We certainly need not assume that MK has a direct route available for repetition; in general his performance levels in spoken word definition correspond closely to his accuracy in word repetition. There is no evidence to suggest that he can repeat words that he cannot understand. Thus we have no grounds for assuming that MK has a 'direct route' for repetition available; it is surely impaired (because word repetition is impaired), but we cannot conclusively demonstrate that it is completely abolished.

At what level is the semantic repetition routine impaired? We have already demonstrated that MK has difficulties in the auditory input lexicon and in the process of access to semantics. The output processes from the semantic system are those also used in picture naming. MK's naming is, in contrast to his very poor repetition, close to normal. Thus we have no grounds for suspecting an impairment in a phonological output lexicon or in access to it; there may, however, be a minor difficulty in output from the semantic system.

Routines available for writing to dictation

In this model of lexical processing, writing nonwords to dictation depends on first converting an input auditory representation by sublexical auditory-to-phonological conversion into an output phonological representation, and then, by the process of sublexical phonological-to-graphemic conversion, generating a graphemic output representation. We have shown that sublexical auditory-to-phonological conversion is not possible for MK— hence his inability to repeat nonwords. This is sufficient to explain his complete failure in writing nonwords to dictation. We in fact have some information to indicate that sublexical phonological-to-orthographic conversion is possible. This is because a substantial proportion of his spelling errors are phonologically plausible renderings of the target word. The occurrence of spelling errors of just the same kind in spontaneous writing by normal people (Hotopf 1980; Wing and Baddeley 1980) is the primary motivation for postulating this link in the model (see Morton 1980a; Ellis 1982; Patterson 1986).

Whether the lexical mapping between the phonological output lexicon and the orthographic output lexicon is also intact is much harder to establish. This route was first postulated to explain the occurrence of substitution of homophones in writing (Morton 1980a); where the homophones substituted have an unusual spelling for that sound pattern, such errors cannot be accounted for by sublexical phonological-to-graphemic conversion. So the existence of the lexical mapping is used to explain substitution of THERE by THEIR (a very common error in normal writing). The only evidence we have regarding this lexical mapping from POL → GOL in MK is a single error: 'paw' written as CLAUSE, which appears to be a homophone error superimposed on a semantic error. The obvious explanation of this is that MK addressed a POL entry as an intermediate stage in generating the output. To the extent that we can safely draw conclusions from a single response, this suggests that MK can use the lexical mapping from POL to GOL.

In almost all tasks involving written output MK shows a small but significant disadvantage with longer words; this applies to delayed copying and written naming. In writing to dictation this output disadvantage for longer words is offset by an input disadvantage with shorter words. What underlying deficit could be responsible for this effect?

Analysis of the performance of two Italian patients with defective graphemic output buffers shows that errors occur with longer words (Miceli, Silveri, and Caramazza 1987; Caramazza, Miceli, Villa, and Romani 1987). MK's spelling errors are frequently phonologically plausible renderings of the words; this strongly suggests that he uses output phonological representations in the phonological output buffer to support graphemic representations. We therefore think that MK has a mild degree of impairment to the graphemic output buffer.

The most striking feature of MK's performance in writing to dictation is its similarity with his oral repetition. Errors of the same kinds occur in very similar proportions. Performance is affected by the same variables in the same way (with the sole exception of the word length effect). We therefore think that the same features that underlie the characteristic pattern in word repetition also underlie his writing to dictation. That is, in both tasks MK primarily uses a semantically mediated routine, in which both the auditory input lexicon and the process of semantic access is impaired.

Routines available for reading

MK reads nonwords with reasonable accuracy, but he makes errors particularly with longer words. This shows that the process of sublexical orthographic-to-phonological conversion is available, but does not work perfectly. We have some indications of the level at which this process is breaking down. There is considerable dispute concerning how a sublexical reading routine might operate—is nonword phonology generated by a system of rules relating letters to sounds, or does it instead depend on analogies between the nonwords and real words that are lexically-represented? (for reviews see, e.g., Kay 1985; Henderson 1985). We do not want to enter into the details of that debate here. We note simply that theories of both kinds have to have (at least) three stages in the procedure. First, the written letter sequence must be recognized and parsed into subword constituents. Second, there must be a procedure (of either rule look-up or discovery of lexical analogy) for determining the phonemes that correspond to these orthographic constituents. And third, there must be a process of phonological assembly, which generates a phonological string, which can be used to drive articulatory output. We can try to determine, on the basis of the available evidence, which of these three subprocesses might be defective in MK.

In visual lexical decision MK performs within the normal range. This demonstrates both that the visual input lexicon must be intact and that he is able to accurately recognize written letters. Thus his problem in nonword reading does not lie in recognition of the component letters.

Derouesné and Beauvois (1985) have described a dyslexic patient whose reading of pseudo-homophones is better than his reading of control nonwords. They interpret this effect in terms of a deficit in the processes of nonword phonological assembly; with pseudo-homophones the existing lexical phonological representation facilitates assembly and output of a phonological string. With MK the difficulty with longer nonwords is evident both with pseudo-homophones and control nonwords (see Howard and Franklin 1987 for details). It is unlikely, then, that a deficit in phonological assembly is at fault.

By exclusion, the most likely level of breakdown is in the process of erecting correspondences between orthography and phonology. The longer the nonword, the more complex this process will be and therefore the more prone to error. The rate of error in this process is low, however. MK achieves quite respectable accuracy in reading non-words.

The sublexical reading routine (SLRR) also contributes to MK's reading of real words. He has difficulty in reading irregular words, especially when they are abstract. When irregular words are misread, his errors are most often phonologically plausible. This indicates that he is using a SLRR, when he does not derive the word's phonology lexically.

Imageability affects MK's written word comprehension; we argued that this reflected a defect in access to lexical semantic representations (or that the representations themselves were impaired). Imageability also affects irregular word reading: this strongly implies that MK is using a semantically mediated routine in reading real words.

The model of lexical processing that we are using incorporates a 'direct route' mapping the orthographic input lexicon to the phonological output lexicon. Clearly this 'route' cannot be intact because if it were MK would be able to read all familiar real words correctly. We are left with the same problem that we had in deciding whether MK was using a 'direct route' in word repetition: it is impossible to decide whether a defective 'direct route' is contributing to his word reading, when we have no characterization of the properties of this direct route. Bub, Cancelliere, and Kertesz (1985) suggest that a defective direct route will work better with high than low frequency words; with MK we found that reading errors occurred particularly with very low frequency irregular words. But errors in visual lexical decision also occur with low frequency items; the frequency effect in word reading may be a simple consequence of the fact that some very low frequency words are not represented in MK's orthographic input lexicon. The frequency effect provides no unambiguous evidence that the 'direct route' contributes to MK's reading. In chapter 12 we will argue that the 'direct route' need not be contributing at all to MK's oral reading; his entire performance can be satisfactorily explained as a result of a combination of information from the semantically mediated lexical routine and the SLRR, both of which are defective in characteristic ways that we have described.

An impairment in converting output phonology into auditory input representations

In this book we have not focused on MK's problem in 'phonological-to-auditory conversion'. This is because we have dealt with the evidence for this impairment in detail in an earlier paper (Howard and Franklin 1987), and we explore its consequences for MK's short term memory in another paper (Howard and Franklin 1989). Here we will simply summarize the evidence that MK's system for converting output phonology into input auditory representations is impaired.

First, MK shows no evidence of the existence of a process of 'phonological-to-auditory conversion' in a number of tasks where its use would result in errors:

— In visual lexical decision he shows no significant difference in latency or accuracy between pseudo-homophones and control non-words, or between regular and irregular real words.
— In word definition, he never misdefines a written word as its homophone.
— Although he misreads very irregular words, he shows no particular difficulty in defining them.

In all these tasks, if MK generated an output phonological representation, and then converted it into an input representation, we would expect characteristic errors that reflect phonological recoding. Another 'surface dyslexic' patient, EE, whom we have contrasted with MK, made these errors in all three tasks and performed significantly worse than MK in all three.

Second, MK shows no evidence of being able to use output phonology to access auditory input representations in tasks that require him to use 'phonological-to-auditory conversion':

— Given pairs of nonwords, such as STAWN STAWK, MK is no better than chance in deciding which would sound like a real word when written.
— He performs very poorly in defining pseudo-homophones such as BOTE or TODE.

He is nevertheless good at pronouncing these pseudo-homophones, so his difficulty cannot be due to a problem in attaining an output phonological representation. He is reasonably good at defining the words when they are presented in spoken form, at least when the words involved are concrete. His problem in understanding pseudo-homophones cannot be completely accounted for by deficits in access to semantics from auditory input. Supporting evidence for this was found in a *post hoc* analysis of the factors affecting his success. His ability to read the pseudo-homophones aloud was a function of their length, but his ability to define them was independent of length but related to the visual similarity between the pseudo-homophone and the corresponding real word. The length effects suggest that while he used the (mildly defective) SLRR to read the words aloud, this routine was not used when he defined them. Instead he seems to have relied on 'approximate visual access' to access a meaning from the pseudo-homophones (see Saffran and Marin 1977). His errors support this. In reading the pseudo-homophones aloud, he makes a few phonemic errors (e.g., TRETE → '/trɛt/'), and in definition he will describe a visually (but not necessarily phonologically) similar word (PHITE → 'pale' [i.e., white]).

In these tasks with pseudo-homophones requiring the use of 'phonological-to-auditory conversion', MK performs very poorly. The contrast patient EE performs much better; in both of these tasks he is significantly better than MK (Howard and Franklin 1987). We argued that this double dissociation reflects the fact that 'phonological-to-auditory conversion' is impossible for MK.

In support of this we went on to show that in memory span tasks MK performs in a very similar way to normal subjects in whom 'phonological-to-auditory conversion' is prevented by concurrent articulation. Thus both MK and normal subjects who are articulating irrelevant material perform worse with lists made up of phonologically similar items (e.g., CGTBDP) than with lists made up of dissimilar items (JSHYLR) when they are presented auditorily but not when they are presented visually. When normal subjects do not have to do concurrent articulation, there is an effect of phonological similarity with visual presentation. Baddeley (1986, etc.) in his influential model of 'working memory' interprets this as showing that concurrent

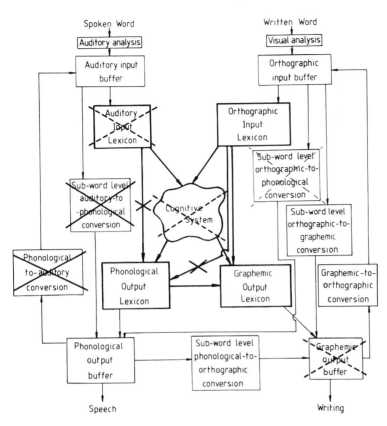

Figure 5
MK's single word processing deficits. A solid cross indicates that a procedure is completely unavailable; a dotted cross, that the procedure still operates for some but not all items and may be responsible for errors.

articulation prevents visually presented material from accessing a phonological input store. MK, in whom 'phonological-to-auditory conversion' is abolished by brain damage, behaves in list memory tasks like a normal subject for whom this process is interfered with by concurrent articulation.

Information converging from several different sources shows that for MK the process of 'phonological-to-auditory conversion' is not available.

Model-based interpretation of deficits: conclusion

By any standards MK's pattern of impairment with single words is complex. By interpreting these in terms of a lexical model, we have nevertheless been able to identify eight different processing impairments which, taken together, can account for his patterns of impairment. These problems vary in their severity: at one extreme we can find no evidence at all for the use of the processes of 'phonological-to-auditory conversion' or for 'sublexical 'auditory-to-phonological conversion', nor have we any conclusive evidence that MK ever uses the 'direct routes' from AIL to POL or from OIL to POL. In figure 5 we therefore mark all four of these processes as abolished. Other of his deficits are major limitations on MK's word recognition and comprehension; the deficit in the auditory input lexicon and the impairment of semantic access or to semantic representations (which affects abstract words more than concrete ones) are both partial. A substantial proportion of items can be processed by these systems.

The other two problems we have identified are, by comparison, minor. While the processes are broadly intact, errors may become apparent with longer words. Thus MK's errors in reading longer nonwords reflect a mild impairment in 'subword level orthographic-to-phonological conversion'. Similarly MK's errors in writing longer words are best accounted for by a mild impairment in holding representations in a graphemic output buffer.

The other processes shown in the model we have been able to show to be intact. We would, of course, be rash to claim that they were completely unimpaired; there may be real impairments which our testing and evaluation was not sensitive enough to detect. Our claim is more modest: the eight problems we have identified, and to some extent characterized, can account for MK's pattern of performance in tasks involving single words.

Chapter 12
Implications for Lexical Theories

The relationship between auditory word recognition and semantics: evidence for top-down processing?

A variety of studies with normal people have demonstrated that semantic and syntactic information from a sentence context can be used to aid auditory word recognition (e.g., Morton 1969; Underwood 1977; Blank and Foss 1978). Studies using Grosjean's (1980) 'gating' method, where a subject is presented with successively larger fragments of a word, demonstrate that top-down context effects can improve the accuracy of word recognition at an early stage; Tyler (1984) shows that context effects can play a role within 100 msec of the start of a word—that is before the whole of the first phoneme has even been heard. Semantic constraints from the context generally have much larger effects than syntactic constraints on the accuracy of word recognition (Tyler and Wessels 1983). Tyler argues that, although top-down processes play an important role in auditory word recognition at an early stage, the process is primarily driven by sensory information; subjects almost always produce responses that are consistent with their auditory input.

In Tyler and Marslen-Wilson's 'cohort model' of auditory word recognition, then, contextual constraints automatically contribute information to auditory word recognition (Marslen-Wilson 1987). Other theoretical perspectives also incorporate mechanisms in which top-down information automatically contributes to word recognition. In McLelland and Elman's (1985) TRACE model of auditory word recognition there is feedback from semantic levels to the word recognition units, just as there is in Morton's logogen model. Within such systems there will be automatic feeding of top-down information to the level of word recognition.

In terms of sensory experience, normal subjects show an extraordinary ability to retrieve a clear percept from degraded phonological information. The most striking demonstration of this is by Warren (1970), who showed that when a phoneme in a word was replaced by white noise, subjects would hear the complete word with a cough in the background.

There are a number of lines of evidence that suggest that MK uses 'top-down' information to aid, and possibly to hinder, auditory word recognition:

— In auditory lexical decision, MK is more likely to miss low imageability words (where his access to semantics is poor) than high imageability words (for which he can retrieve relatively good semantics).

— In repetition and writing to dictation he is more likely to misrecognize a low imageability word as another phonologically related word.

In word-to-picture matching tasks, MK performs extremely well. In Bishop and Byng's (1984) LUVS test, for example, he made no errors at all. This contrasts with a high rate of errors in tasks (such as word definition, or oral repetition) where MK cannot predict in advance the words he is likely to be presented with. These expectations can actually mislead him; in the auditory name judgment task he accepted, and therefore *mis*recognized, 40% of phonological distractors. In doing this, MK is performing abnormally; as Tyler (1984) demonstrates, normal subjects almost always produce auditory word recognition candidates in accordance with the sensory information available. MK, like normal subjects, uses top-down information to aid in auditory word recognition, but because of loss of information in the word specifications in an auditory input lexicon, he is forced to use this information to an unusual extent. With MK, top-down information is able to play a role in processing at the point where he has insufficient information —the auditory input lexicon.

At one point in our argument we claimed that an imageability effect in auditory lexical decision was evidence for the use of top-down semantic information in word recognition. An alternative explanation of this would be that lexical decision is done on the basis of access to semantic representations, rather than at the level of the auditory word recognition system. We think this unlikely for two reasons. First, in visual lexical decision MK performs within the range of Rickard's (1986) normal controls, despite his problem in comprehension of visually presented abstract words. In visual lexical decision, then, MK cannot be making his lexical decisions on the basis of access to semantics; in the visual modality, lexical access alone appears sufficient for lexical decision. It cannot therefore be generally true that MK makes lexical decisions on the basis of access to semantics. Second, not all patients with difficulties in auditory word comprehension require access to semantics for auditory lexical decision. We are currently investigating a patient DRB who, like MK, is much better at understanding concrete words than abstract words with auditory presentation. Unlike MK, DRB's auditory lexical decision is good with both concrete and abstract words. For DRB, then, access to an entry in the auditory input lexicon appears to be sufficient for lexical decision. To be consistent with these findings, we have to suggest that MK makes lexical decisions on the basis of information at a lexical level; the effect of imageability thus provides support for the use of top down information in word recognition.

On the origin of a naming deficit; evidence for the role of a semantic lexicon?

In terms of number of correct responses, MK has only a mild naming impairment; in standardized tests his scores hover around the lower edge of the range for normal subjects. Yet qualitatively his performance is disturbed: he makes a high rate of semantic errors. There is striking similarity between his spoken and written naming:

— Error rates are very similar.
— The types of errors are very similar.
— The same items attract errors in the two tasks.

The primary source of MK's naming errors is semantic, in that the majority of errors are semantically related. If the semantic representations themselves were impaired, this would result in an equivalent problem is spoken and written naming. However, from MK's performance in the 'Pyramid and Palm Trees' test, we were able to deduce that from a picture input MK was able to access conceptual and lexical semantic representations, which were reasonably accurate. His naming errors, in contrast, reflect the use of only partial semantic information. We argued that therefore MK's difficulty in naming could most appropriately be described as *an output semantic deficit.* Many theories of word retrieval view the processes of output from the semantic system as modality specific; in Morton's (1980a) 'logogen model', for instance, the addressing of the phonological output lexicon and the addressing of the graphemic output lexicon from the 'cognitive system' are entirely independent processes. In this system, the similarities between MK's spoken and written naming is due to two independent information processing impairments, which just happen to be qualitatively similar.

A number of authors, operating with different kinds of evidence, have suggested that word retrieval is a two-stage process (e.g., Butterworth 1980; Garrett 1980; Kempen and Huijbers 1983; Levelt and Maassen 1981; see Butterworth 1987, for a review). Butterworth suggests that a central semantic representation is used to access an entry in a 'semantic lexicon', where entries are organized in terms of semantic similarity. Entries in this semantic lexicon then yield an address that can be used to access the corresponding entries in an output lexicon, which is organized in terms of phonological similarity. This kind of system is therefore able to account for two types of errors in speech production: misaddressing at the level of the semantic lexicon results in semantically related real word errors, and misaddressing at the phonological output lexicon results in phonologically related real word errors (Butterworth 1980). One important property of the semantic lexicon is that it is *intermodal*; in both written and spoken word production the semantic lexicon must be accessed prior to word retrieval from either of the two output lexicons. And, in input, the semantic lexicon intervenes between word recognition in the input lexicons and access to the semantic system. A possible architecture of this system is illustrated in figure 6.

Butterworth et al. (1984) suggested that a semantic lexicon deficit could explain the occurrence of some semantic errors in aphasic naming (see also Howard et al. 1985; Howard 1985a). Where a patient retrieves a full and complete central semantic representation but misaddresses entries in an output lexicon, semantically related real word errors will result. Because the semantic lexicon is involved in retrieval of both spoken and written words, the same error pattern should emerge in either modality of naming.

A semantic lexicon can therefore account for output semantic errors qualitatively and quantitatively identical in spoken and written naming. Theories in which addressing of the two output lexicons is entirely separate will have to view MK's naming problems as due to two different lesions. The theories therefore make very different kinds of predictions: if there is a semantic lexicon it will be impossible to have a semantic level of deficit specific to one modality. In Morton's 'logogen model', output semantic

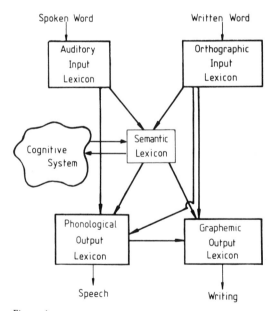

Figure 6
A semantic lexicon that intervenes between semantic representations and input and output lexicons.

deficits will be modality-specific; one would therefore predict that there will be dissociations at a semantic level between spoken and written naming.

MK's naming provides the first clear-cut case of an output semantic naming impairment that is independent of modality of naming. He can access, for use in comprehension tasks, a much more accurate lexical-semantic representation than he is able to use in word retrieval. We suggest, then, that MK may have two different kinds of semantic-level problem. Semantic errors in output do not seem to be sensitive to abstractness and could be attributed to misaddressing at the level of the semantic lexicon. The problem in input, in contrast, is less marked than in output (at least with picturable items) and is sensitive to stimulus words' abstractness.

Orthographic errors in oral picture naming: Evidence for a graphemic-to-orthographic conversion system?

In oral naming, with pictures whose names have an irregular spelling-to-sound correspondence, MK sometimes produces a spoken name that is very much like his reading response for that word, one that, in fact, is a phonologically plausible rendering of the spelling. Thus, for example, he named a COMB as '/kɒmb/' and a BEAR as '/bɪə/', which for him would be characteristic reading responses for these same items. Although relatively rare in absolute numbers, these orthographically based errors make up a very high proportion of the phonologically related errors that MK makes in naming pictures with irregularly spelled names; they cannot be accounted for as phonological errors which, by chance, correspond to the words' orthography. Similar errors are found, although relatively infrequently, in oral word repetition.

The occurrence of these errors demonstrates that MK sometimes uses orthographic word specifications to generate spoken naming responses. In the model in figure 1, we incorporated a routine of 'graphemic-to-orthographic conversion' that is needed to account for these errors. Our account of the source of these errors is as follows:

(i) MK fails to retrieve a phonological word form from the phonological output lexicon.

(ii) He retrieves an orthographic word form from the graphemic output lexicon.

(iii) This is transferred into the graphemic output buffer and then is processed by 'graphemic-to-orthographic conversion' into an input orthographic code.

(iv) He generates the phonology for this code using the 'sublexical orthographic-to-phonological conversion' system. This yields a phonologically plausible error.

The occurrence of these errors provides one line of evidence for the existence of a system for conversion of output graphemic codes into input orthographic codes (see Howard and Franklin 1987 for further discussion). Converging evidence for the existence of this conversion system comes from a study of repetition priming by Monsell (1987b). He showed that writing a word, without being able to see it, primes subsequent visual lexical decision. He interprets this as evidence for a system relating output graphemic representations to input orthography.

The relationship between 'semantic errors in repetition' and 'deep dysgraphia': Evidence for one form of lexical organization?

Within the model of lexical processing that we set out in the introduction, two of the routines available for writing words to dictation are dependent on retrieving an output phonological representation as an intermediate stage (see figure 4). Thus the sublexical writing routine involves using the 'sublexical auditory-to-phonological conversion system' followed by a 'sublexical phonological-to-graphemic conversion system'. The non-semantic lexical routine involves accessing a word form in the auditory input lexicon and using this to address an entry in the phonological output lexicon, which in turn addresses the graphemic output lexicon.

In this system the two nonsemantic routines for writing to dictation are partly dependent on the corresponding oral repetition routines. As a consequence, where either the sublexical routine or the nonsemantic lexical routine is unavailable for repetition, it will also be unavailable for writing to dictation. This generates a straightforward prediction; all patients who rely on a semantic routine in oral word repetition will also rely on a semantic routine for writing to dictation, and so all patients who make semantic errors in repetition will also make semantic errors in writing to dictation.

Note that the converse does not hold; this system predicts that semantic errors in writing to dictation can be dissociated from semantic errors in repetition. Thus a patient might be able to repeat nonwords using an intact sublexical repetition routine, but be unable to write them to dictation because of a failure in 'sublexical phonological-to-graphemic conversion'; this probably applies to Bub and Kertesz's (1982) patient JC.

This form of lexical organization is not the only possible arrangement. Some authors (e.g., Ellis, 1982) have assumed that there can be direct lexical addressing of output orthography from auditory input, without intermediate output phonological coding. In a model of this kind, the lexical nonsemantic routine for repetition is entirely independent of the corresponding routines for writing to dictation. There is no necessary association of semantic errors in repetition and writing to dictation; in fact, there is no reason not to expect complete dissociation.

In a careful review of the evidence, Patterson (1986) argues that there is no evidence available for direct addressing; she prefers the theory where writing to dictation depends on repetition routines, because the existence of all the processing systems can be motivated independently by evidence for other sources. This view predicts, then, that all patients who make semantic errors in repetition will show a very similar pattern of impairment in writing to dictation to the one shown in word repetition. As we demonstrated the similarities for MK are extremely close:

— Accuracy in writing to dictation is very similar to accuracy in oral word repetition.
— Both repetition and writing to dictation are affected by the same variables (see table 34).
— The same types of errors occur with very similar frequencies in the two tasks (see table 35).

The evidence reviewed in the introduction supports the view that *all* patients who make semantic errors in repetition have exactly the same kind of problem in writing to dictation. While evidence from *associations* is inevitably weak (it takes only one case report to show that there can be a *dissociation*), this supports Patterson's (1986) view of the functional architecture of the systems available for writing to dictation.

Two sources of evidence for separate auditory input and phonological output lexicons

The earliest versions of the 'logogen model' postulated only a single lexicon serving both recognition and production of phonological and orthographic word forms (e.g., Morton, 1964, 1969). Then, in response to evidence that showed that auditory word recognition does not prime visual word recognition, and conversely visual word recognition does not prime auditory word recognition (Winnick and Daniel 1970; Clarke and Morton 1983), Morton (1979, 1980a) revised the model to separate the single lexicon into the four separate lexicons shown in figure 1.

In 1981, Allport and Funnell criticized Morton's position; they argued that the priming data motivated the distinction between orthographic and phonological lexicons but did not force the separation into separate input and output forms. In a series of publications, Funnell (1983b; Coltheart and Funnell 1987) and Allport (1983, 1984a) have continued to argue that all the available data can be accounted for by phonological and orthographic lexicons serving both as word recognition devices and as sources of word specifications for production. Other authors have attempted to accumulate evidence for the separation of input and output lexicons from studies of priming (e.g., Monsell 1985, 1987a, 1987b), or of dual tasks (e.g., Shallice, McLeod, and Lewis 1984), but the results have not proved conclusive either way.

Allport and Funnell accept that there are separate phonological and orthographic lexicons. Allport (1983) argues that one particular piece of neuropsychological evidence provides a conclusive demonstration of this. He observes that 'deep dyslexic' patients make semantic errors in oral word reading, and continues:

> The preservation of meaning from target word to spoken response ... confirms that the written word for which the patient cannot generate the correct spoken form, nevertheless must have succeeded in evoking some representation of its meaning.... The important point for our argument, however, is that the *written words must evoke work-meanings without being able to evoke the corresponding spoken word form.* This combination—of inability to derive a phonological representation of a written word, while successfully evoking its meaning—is direct evidence both for the independent representation of [spoken and] written word forms *and* for their independent access to word meanings.   (pp. 80–81; original italics)

Allport argues that the written word had successfully been recognized, because this is a necessary precondition for retrieving its meaning. Yet the occurrence of semantic errors indicates that the spoken word form had not been accessed; the (unaccessed) spoken word form must therefore be different from the (accessed) written word form.

The same argument, in exactly the same form, can be applied to the occurrence of semantic errors in single word repetition: the errors indicate that a word has been correctly recognized from auditory input, but the corresponding spoken word form was not produced. If they were in a single lexicon then, when a word's meaning is available, its output phonology should also be available. Thus Allport's argument shows that semantic errors in repetition constitute strong, or even conclusive, evidence for separate input and output phonological lexicons.

There is one way in which semantic repetition errors might be accounted for in terms of a single phonological lexicon that is used in both input and output. Allport's (1983) argument assumes that each lexical entry will have a single output threshold, so that when an auditorily presented word is recognized, both its spoken form and its central semantic representation become available. One could, however, adopt a position that Morton (1968) put forward to account for semantic errors in reading in the single logogen model. He suggested that the logogen could have two independent output mechanisms, one to semantics and one to output phonology, which have independent output thresholds. Suppose also that some entries have raised thresholds for phonological output, but normal thresholds for output to semantics. With these items, the patient will be able to retrieve the corresponding meaning, without being able to produce a spoken word form; in order to produce some response, the patient will be forced to retrieve another semantically related phonological word form whose threshold is not abnormally raised.[12]

This account is admittedly *ad hoc*. It also suffers from two more serious criticisms. First, it is not at all clear what are the computational consequences of postulating two separate output thresholds in a 'single' lexicon. There is a real possibility that this 'single lexicon' account becomes merely a notational variant of the theory of separate input and output lexicons. Second, once separate output thresholds are accepted, there is no good reason not to return to a single lexicon subserving phonological and orthographic word recognition and production, with multiple thresholds for outputs of different kinds. This would, in effect, be a return to Morton's (1969) version of the single 'logogen model'. There certainly is no principled reason for accepting a division into separate orthographic and phonological lexicons, and then denying that evidence of precisely the same kind can motivate a distinction between separate input and output lexicons for phonology.

A second kind of evidence from MK's behavior also favors separate input and output lexicons. In discussing this issue, Allport (1984a) points out that a theory with separate input and output lexicons will allow for selective impairment of one of the lexicons. He goes on to argue that there is no neuropsychological evidence for this kind of *dissociation*. In a subsequent paper he tries to show that, on the contrary, there is a necessary *association* between phonological errors in speech production (for example in repetition, reading, or naming) and acceptance of closely related phonological distractors in judging the appropriate name for a picture (in effect, our picture name judgment task; Allport 1984b). He claims that this co-occurrence is strong evidence that, when the phonological lexicon is degraded, errors of the same kind will occur in both speech production and comprehension.

Like Allport's patients, MK accepted phonologically related distractors in the name judgment task; he makes errors in lexical decision and misrecognizes words in repetition and writing to dictation. We have argued that this difficulty reflects a loss of distinctiveness in representations in the

---

12. In this case, one might predict that semantic errors would be higher in word frequency (and so more easily elicited) than the words that give rise to the errors. As we showed in the analyses, there were no word frequency differences between semantic error responses and their stimuli.

auditory input lexicon; we were able to show that this could not be attributed to a deficit in phonemic perception or in hearing, but did reflect a lexical deficit.

This lexical deficit is really rather severe; in the name judgment task MK accepted 40% of phonologically related distractors each of which differed in a single phoneme. This suggests that for each phoneme, on only 60% of occasions does he have a phonological specification which can reliably distinguish the phoneme from another. If the same kind of impairment were to be evident in name production, MK should have only a 60% chance of producing each individual phoneme correctly; speech production should be seriously phonologically disturbed. When we tested this, by asking MK to name the pictures whose names had been involved in the name judgment task, MK made just two phoneme errors in one hundred items. Since the average length of these words was about 5 phonemes, he has approximately a 0.4% probability that a phoneme specification is not correct.

There is, therefore, a massive disparity between the incidence of phonologically related errors in auditory word recognition and phonological word production of precisely the kind that Allport (1984a) predicts, on the basis of his theoretical position, should not exist. MK, in fact, demonstrates degraded phonological specifications for auditory word recognition and intact (or very much less degraded) phonological specifications for spoken word production. This dissociation is consistent only with separate input and output lexicons for phonological word forms. There is only one way that we can see to reconcile this result with the proposal of a single phonological lexicon for input and output. This is to claim that there is impairment in the process of lexical access at a level which our tests of phonological processing could not detect rather than degraded representations in the lexicon itself. This proposal could save the theory of a single lexicon, but at the cost of postulating a new level of impairment for which we have no direct evidence. We prefer to follow Allport's (1984a) suggestion that minimal pair judgments can be used to assess the intactness of prelexical representations, but that auditory lexical decision and picture name judgments require the use of lexical phonological representations. Allport points out that "the hypothesis of a *single* inventory of phonological word-forms employed in both reception and production enjoys the advantage not only of theoretical parsimony but also of an attractive empirical vunerability. Even a single patient, in whom selective, dissociated impairment of either receptive or expressive phonological word-forms could be unambiguously demonstrated, would threaten to disprove it" (Allport, 1984a, p225).

MK, we think, is such a patient. His patterns of impairment are apparently incompatible with Allport's hypothesis.

Imageability and regularity effects in oral word reading: Evidence for the interaction of information from lexical and nonlexical routines?

MK often reads words with irregular spelling-to-sound correspondences correctly; in these cases he cannot be relying exclusively on a 'sublexical' reading routine, but must be using lexically derived information. We argued in chapter 11 that the 'direct route' from the visual input lexicon to the phonological output lexicon is certainly defective; indeed there is no evidence that he ever uses information from a nonsemantic lexical routine. His semantic reading routine is more intact for concrete words than for abstract ones. We therefore predicted that the semantic reading routine would be more likely to provide useful, word-specific information for concrete words than abstract words; the effect of spelling-to-sound regularity on oral word reading should therefore be more marked with low imageability words. This prediction was confirmed; MK was very accurate in reading both regular and irregular high imageability words but was very much worse at reading low imageability irregular words than their matched regular low imageability controls. This pattern confirms that MK's lexical reading routine is impaired at a semantic level.

MK achieves impressive accuracy in reading high imageability irregular words. How does he do it? We showed in the written picture name judgment task that MK does not reliably access the complete and correct semantics from written words: he is liable to accept a close contrast coordinate as a correct name for a picture. Furthermore, as shown in his picture naming, MK makes semantic errors in the process of output from the semantic system. If, in oral reading, he could only rely on a loose semantic specification for word retrieval, he would make semantic errors in reading, even with concrete words. These are not found: MK *never* makes phonologically unrelated semantic errors in oral word reading. Therefore he cannot be relying exclusively on this (defective) semantic routine in reading, even with concrete words.

It is also clear that he cannot be relying exclusively on information from a sublexical reading routine when he reads concrete words aloud. If he did, there would be a regularity effect, and in fact we would expect him to read all irregularly spelled words incorrectly. But, as we demonstrated, there is no regularity effect in concrete word reading.

Since MK cannot be relying exclusively on either the semantic reading routine or the sublexical reading routine, he must be using a *combination* of information from the two routines in word reading (cf. Howard 1985a; Margolin et al. 1985). In reviewing the evidence on the contribution of lexical and nonlexical routines in oral reading by normal subjects, Patterson and Coltheart (1987) suggest that instead of competition between the routines (as, e.g., in Forster and Chambers' 1973 or Coltheart's 1978 'horse race' models), there may be *combination* of information (cf. Scheerer 1987). MK provides persuasive neuropsychological evidence for this view; where neither the semantic nor the sublexical reading routine is able to guarantee a correct response by itself, they are able to combine to ensure a high level of performance.

The notion of combining information from the two processing routines can explain why MK does not make semantic errors in reading. Given that the semantic system is degraded, a range of semantically related word forms in the output lexicon, which includes the correct word, will receive some activation (cf. Howard and Orchard-Lisle 1984). For words with a regular spelling-to-sound correspondence, the sublexical routine will provide information that is consistent with the correct response, which will be one of the phonological forms receiving activation from the semantic routine. With this combined activation, the correct word form will be very likely to be produced. Production of semantic errors will never be supported by the sublexical route, so there will never be sufficient activation for them to be produced. There will be less support from the sublexical routine for words with irregular spelling-to-sound correspondence. As the words become more irregular, there will be less and less sublexical support; mildly irregular words will be more likely to be read correctly than those with very unusual relationships between spelling and sound. This then provides a natural account of the effect of 'degree of regularity' on MK's reading, which could be extended to other surface dyslexic patients who show a similar effect (cf. Shallice, Warrington, and McCarthy 1983; Kay and Lesser 1985).

The demonstration of interaction between reading routines has some important implications. Schwartz, Saffran, and Marin (1980) and Funnel (1983a) argue that their patients provide conclusive evidence for the existence of a nonsemantic lexical reading routine. In both cases, they demonstrate that the patients have access only to partial semantic information from written words; they make comprehension errors in tasks involving closely related semantic distractors, but they can read (some or most) irregularly spelled words correctly. On these grounds they assume that a semantically based routine, because it is not working perfectly, cannot be providing *any* lexically specific information in oral word reading; word-specific phonological information must then be derived from another non-semantic lexical routine—a 'direct' connection between the orthographic input lexicon and the phonological output lexicon.

The key assumption in this argument is that, if the semantic routine is not working perfectly, it can be contributing no useful information; our data from MK demonstrate that the assumption is false. These two neuro-psychological cases do not provide strong evidence in favor of the existence of a 'direct' lexical reading routine. Other kinds of evidence may prove more persuasive in establishing whether there is a 'direct route' for word reading; assessing this issue in general is beyond the scope of the present work. Any neuropsychological evidence on this issue will, however, have to take into account the ways in which different sources of *partial* information can interact in producing a response.

Morphological errors

MK makes substantial numbers of errors in repeating or writing to dictation words with inflectional or derivational affixes, but not in reading them aloud. The most common type of error is omission of the suffix, or substitution of an incorrect suffix. Errors of this kind can be hard to interpret. MK makes semantic errors and phonologically related errors not involving affixes. Since morphological errors result in a response that is closely related to the stimulus both semantically and phonologically, it is possible that they are mixed errors caused by a combination of the factors that result in semantic and phonological errors (cf. Shallice and McGill 1978). We were able to show that MK is significantly more likely to make an error in repetition or writing to dictation with words with inflectional suffixes than those with derivational suffixes; in both cases the majority of his errors are suffix omissions. Thus he is more likely to repeat or write 'draining' as 'drain' than to produce 'drainage' as 'drain'. There is approximately equal visual and semantic similarity between the inflected and derived forms and the root. MK's difficulty with inflected words must therefore result from a particular deficit in processing inflected words. However, we remain unclear about the source of his affix errors with derived words; these might reflect a genuine difficulty in processing the derivational suffixes, or they might simply be errors resulting from the combination of visual and semantic similarity between the stimulus and response. At present we do not have the data to choose between these explanations.

Miceli and Caramazza (1988) offer an account of an Italian patient FS who makes a very high rate of inflectional errors in single word repetition; derivational errors also occur but are very much less frequent. His repetition resembles MK's in two further ways:

— FS's nonword repetition is very poor (10% correct).
— 'Content' words are repeated better than 'function' words (when list imageability is not controlled).

There are very striking differences:

— For FS nonmorphological errors are very rare: semantic errors make up less than 1% of errors, and phonologically related real words only 2%.

— Repetition is better for short words than long words, and better for high frequency words than low frequency words (although it is not clear whether imageability was controlled in the relevant tests).

Miceli and Caramazza provide no information on the effects of imageability on FS's repetition, nor any data on writing to dictation. But they do show that FS makes a high rate of morphological errors in spontaneous speech and speculate that these errors may have the same cause as morphological errors in repetition. If there is a common cause, it constrains the locus of the inflectional errors to the processes of output from the semantic system.

MK's spontaneous speech is very different from FS's. It is fluent, with a wide variety of grammatical constructions. There are some syntactically unacceptable sentences in his spontaneous speech (i.e., 'paragrammatisms'; see Butterworth and Howard 1987), but these sentences are infrequent. In appendix 2 we present the transcription of MK's spoken account of the story of Cinderella. A number of different kinds of paragrammatisms occur, and his speech is clearly hindered by retrieval difficulties for both main verbs and nouns. The complete analysis of his speech is not relevant here, but we should note that there are many appropriately used inflections. For example:

The two women wanted to have good shoes
She didn't have a drink but she liked it just the same
I forget what these things are

In only two cases is there clear evidence of omission or addition of a suffix:

And then she pick it up
She get a nice places for her

So while MK omits inflectional and derivational affixes at a high rate in repetition and writing to dictation, he rarely omits them in spontaneous speech. This clearly suggests that MK's difficulty with suffixed words lies in the process of access to central representations in the cognitive system. Since in MK both repetition and writing to dictation depend on access to the semantic system, this would explain the similarity in performance with affixed words in these tasks.

MK has a very severe deficit in the comprehension of spoken and written sentences (Howard and Franklin 1988). This applies to sentences where comprehension depends on correct analysis of the structural information carried by inflections and free-standing function words. But it also applies to sentences where correct comprehension could be achieved simply on the basis of the linear order of the content words, ignoring all structural information from inflections or function words. Thus MK's sentence comprehension deficit cannot be attributed to an input impairment in processing grammatical morphemes, since there seems to be a more general difficulty in comprehension of structured sentences. It is tempting, however, to ascribe his sentence comprehension problems and his difficulties in repetition and writing to dictation with inflected words and function words to a common underlying cause—an impairment to a syntactic parser that analyses input. Under this view MK would also make inflectional errors in reading aloud, were he not able to generate the correct phonology via his sublexical reading routine.

The difference between inflectional and derivational suffixes we find more predictable. In general inflections carry information that plays a syntactic role and has a constant interpretation, while derivations have a meaning that varies according to the stem to which it is attached (see Aronoff 1976). A parsing procedure might therefore strip inflectional suffixes from words in order to determine the structure of the sentence. A defective parser would therefore result in loss of inflectional and not derivational suffixes.

The contrast between FS and MK suggests that there can be at least two different levels of breakdown in repetition of inflected words. FS's problem is most plausibly attributed to a difficulty in producing the correct affixes in output, while MK's seems to reflect an impairment in structural processing of inflections in input.

High imageability and low imageability words

In almost every task illustrated in table 34, MK performs better with high imageability words than low imageability words. Why?

We suggested that this demonstrated that MK was operating with lexical semantic information which was, in some way, defective. In other patients we find the same pattern of better performance with high imageability than low imageability words, in every case where there are semantic errors in the task. This applies to semantic errors in reading ('deep dyslexia'; Coltheart, Patterson, and Marshall 1980), writing to dictation ('deep dysgraphia'; Bub and Kertesz 1982), and in repetition. Greater vulnerability of abstract rather than concrete word meanings may be a very general feature among aphasic patients. We have recently been studying the patterns of breakdown in comprehension in fluent aphasic patients; the only feature that all these subjects have in common is a difficulty in comprehension of low imageability words (Franklin 1989).

It is at least plausible to claim that when the lexical semantic system is impaired, abstract words are more vulnerable than concrete ones. But it is more complex than that: Warrington (1975) describes a (demented) patient AB who was very much better at defining spoken abstract words than concrete ones, and Warrington (1981) reports another patient who was very much better at reading abstract words than concrete ones. It appears that semantics for abstract words can sometimes be much less impaired than for concrete words.

An explanation would appear to be restricted to one of two general possibilities: differences in storage of concrete and abstract semantic information, or differences in systems that manipulate a single kind of semantic information. A number of proposals have been made of the first kind; Allport (1985) suggests that the meaning of concrete words may be expressed primarily in terms of distributed representations of sensory features, which will not be vulnerable to localized lesions, because the information is distributed across the cortex (cf. Funnell and Allport, 1987).[13] Warrington and Shallice (1984) suggest separate storage of sensory and functional semantic information. We have already suggested that MK's problem in abstract word comprehension may not be paralleled by a corresponding difficulty in abstract word production. In Warrington and Shallice's theory this could easily be accommodated as a problem in access to abstract word semantics, with no impairment to the semantic system itself. The second kind of proposal has been advanced by Howard (1985a). Here lexical semantic information (which is of a single kind) can be used in two different ways: the 'sensory-imaginal system' creates and manipulates information in the form of images, and the 'propositional reasoning system' operates deductive reasoning systems on semantic information. In a system of this kind, a difficulty with abstract words would not necessarily be attributed to a loss of semantic information but rather, as Goldstein (1948) originally suggested, to a difficulty in using lexical semantic information in tasks requiring manipulation of abstract information.

The data we have obtained from MK does not allow us to distinguish between these different explanations. It is empirically clear that MK has a quite general difficulty in tasks requiring him to use semantic information derived from low imageability (abstract) words.

13. An account of this kind does not appear to be able to deal with patients like Warrington's (1975), where comprehension is more impaired for concrete words than abstract words.

Chapter 13
Symptomcomplexes

Levels of breakdown in auditory comprehension: a revision of the concept of 'word deafness'

We have shown that MK has a deficit in word comprehension that is much more severe when words are presented auditorily rather than visually. In this sense, MK's comprehension difficulties are (partly) modality-specific and therefore legitimately described as 'word deafness'.

Traditional conceptions of 'word deafness' have distinguished between 'word sound deafness' and 'word meaning deafness'. As we discussed in the introduction, in word sound deafness patients show difficulties in perception of speech sounds, despite normal hearing. Performance is poor in phoneme categorization and in minimal pair judgments. In word meaning deafness, words are correctly perceived, and often correctly repeated, but the patient is unable to access their meaning. In just three cases—those reported by Bramwell (1897), Morton (1980a), and Kohn and Friedman's (1986) patient HN—there is clear evidence that a heard word must have accessed the correct input lexicon entry, because one or more irregularly spelled words were written correctly without comprehension.

MK represents a third level of impairment in auditory word comprehension, which has not been systematically described before. His primary difficulty is in word specification in an auditory input lexicon. Prelexical word sound discrimination is intact, and semantic factors play a role only because of 'top-down processes'. This problem could accurately be described as 'word form deafness'.

To summarize: three varieties of 'word deafness' can be distinguished by their levels of breakdown. In 'word meaning deafness', the impairment is in the process of postlexical semantic access: word comprehension is impaired, and the deficit is specific to auditory input, but auditory lexical decision, phoneme minimal pair judgments, and hearing are intact. In 'word form deafness', the impairment is in the auditory input lexicon: there is an auditory word comprehension impairment and a deficit in auditory lexical decision, but minimal pair judgments and hearing are intact. In 'word sound deafness', the impairment is in prelexical speech sound analysis; auditory word comprehension, auditory lexical decision, and minimal pair judgments are all disturbed, but hearing is normal for nonspeech sounds.

'Semantic errors in repetition': a provisional summary of a symptomcomplex

MK makes semantic errors in single word repetition. In addition, his single word repetition shows the following features:

(i)   Nonword repetition is impossible.
(ii)   Repetition is better for concrete words than abstract words.
(iii)   Repetition is better for unaffixed words than affixed words.
(iv)   Repetition is better for long words than short words.
(iv)   Phonologically related real word errors,
(v)   morphologically related errors, and
(vi)   unrelated real word errors occur.

We argued that MK uses a semantic routine in oral word repetition. We argued that a sublexical routine was not available, and as a result MK could not repeat nonwords. The reason for this difficulty can be pinpointed; he has no difficulty in holding input nonword auditory representations, as in, for example, nonword minimal pair judgments. He has little or no difficulty in generating and producing nonword output phonological representations, as shown by his ability to read nonwords aloud with reasonable accuracy. His impairment must therefore lie in the process of converting input auditory codes to output phonological codes in units smaller than whole known words—that is, in the process of 'sublexical auditory-to-phonological conversion'.

There is also positive evidence that MK uses a semantic routine for repetition. He makes semantic errors, and success in repetition is affected by a semantic variable—the word's imageability. Thus he cannot be using a nonsemantic lexical routine for repetition.

MK clearly makes morphological errors in repetition; whether he does so depends strongly on the type of suffix on the stimulus word. He is much more likely to delete an inflection than a derivation. This shows that these errors are not simply phonological and/or semantic errors, but, with inflectional suffixes at least, they involve a genuine morphological component. The inflected word 'draining', and the derived word 'drainage' are very close both phonologically and semantically to the root form 'drain'. But MK is much more likely to repeat 'drainage' than 'draining' correctly, and much more likely to omit the '-ing' than the '-age'.

Every patient who makes semantic errors in reading also makes morphological errors, especially with suffixed words (see Coltheart, Patterson, and Marshall 1980). This applies both with patients who are agrammatic in speech production and those who are not. This co-occurrence between semantic and morphological errors has led some authors to suggest that, in reading, a semantic routine by itself may be unable to support correct reading of inflections (e.g., Patterson 1982). Why this might be remains unclear. Our finding of the same association between semantic errors and morphological errors in repetition suggests that, in repetition also, the occurrence of inflectional errors may be attributable to MK's reliance on a (defective) semantic routine in repetition.

In this view, therefore, failure in nonword repetition, the imageability effect, and morphological errors all reflect reliance on a (defective) semantic repetition routine; we would therefore claim that all of these features will occur along with semantic errors in repetition.

MK cannot use a sublexical or nonsemantic lexical repetition routine. His semantic routine is defective in three different ways: he has a deficit in phonological specifications in the input lexicon (we argued above that this was responsible for his better repetition of long words than short words); he has a deficit in semantic access, which is more marked with abstract words than concrete words (this is responsible for the imageability effect in repetition); he has an output semantic deficit (which is probably the source of some, or even all, of MK's semantic errors in repetition).

If the semantic routine were working perfectly, we would expect that all real words would be repeated perfectly (except that synonym substitution errors might occur). The occurrence of semantic errors indicates that it is not. Therefore we would expect that any patient who makes semantic errors in repetition will show the characteristics of reliance on a defective semantic routine. We would therefore predict that features (i) and (ii) (failure with nonwords and imageability effect), and possibly (iii) and (v) (difficulty with suffixed words, and morphological errors) in the list above, have the same cause as the semantic errors. The other features of MK's reading impairment (the length effect, and phonologically related errors) have a separate cause, and we would expect them to dissociate from semantic errors in repetition.

The data from patients who make semantic errors in repetition that we assembled in the introduction support this view. Where information is available, all the patients show an imageability effect, an inability to repeat nonwords, and (with two possible exceptions) morphological errors. On the other hand only Michel's patient MR shows MK's superiority with long words compared with short words; in fact Goldblum's (1980) patients BF and MAL show a length effect in the opposite direction. And phonologically related real word errors are only reported in two subjects (BF and MAL).

This provides some evidence to support our view that there are a set of symptoms that will co-occur with semantic errors, all of which reflect reliance on a defective semantic routine for oral word repetition.

MK's reading problem: a 'central' surface dyslexia?

With MK, as with other surface dyslexics, two phenomena demonstrate that he sometimes (or often) has to rely on a 'sublexical orthographic-to-phonological conversion' system in reading real words aloud. First, he is better at reading words with regular spelling-to-sound correspondences than those with irregular correspondences; second, a high proportion of his reading errors are phonologically plausible renderings of the letter string. That he has to rely on a 'sublexical' routine for real word reading demonstrates that the lexical reading routines must in some way be defective.

The earlier descriptions of 'surface dyslexics' were of patients who, apart from their difficulty in reading irregular words aloud, also had difficulty in understanding irregular words (and regular words with homophones) (e.g., Marshall and Newcombe 1973; Coltheart, Masterson, Byng, Prior, and Riddoch 1983). This pattern of performance was taken to demonstrate that these subjects had to use a phonological code (derived via a 'sublexical routine') for semantic access. The implication was that the lexical reading routines had broken down at the level of the 'orthographic input lexicon'; as a result, lexical decision and semantic access could not rely on direct visual word recognition, but instead the patients had to use phonological recoding.

In this traditional pattern of surface dyslexia, the lexical routines break down due to impairment of the orthographic input lexicon; so it can be described as 'input surface dyslexia'. But any point of breakdown in lexical reading routines should be sufficient to cause 'surface dyslexic' reading—provided that the 'sublexical' routine is still functional. A number of authors have suggested that there will be a second class of patient—'output surface dyslexics'—where the deficit is at the level of the phonological output lexicon (see Patterson, Marshall, and Coltheart 1985). Here, word comprehension and visual lexical decision will be normal for all types of words, but the patient will not be able to produce the correct spoken response because of missing information in an output lexicon; evidence of the output lexicon deficit should also be available in other, nonreading tasks—the patient should show a word retrieval deficit in naming or spontaneous speech. Although this theoretical pattern has been predicted, none of the patients who have been described so far fulfills this pattern with any precision; as described, all the candidate patients have rather severely disturbed written word comprehension problems, which, where it has been properly tested, can be shown to depend on the regularity of the words' spelling-to-sound relationship.

A third pattern of 'surface dyslexia' is possible, where the nonsemantic lexical reading routine (the 'direct route' from the orthographic input lexicon to the phonological output lexicon) is not available, and the semantic lexical routine breaks down because of impairment(s) at a central, semantic level, while the orthographic input lexicon and the phonological output lexicon remain intact.[14] Visual lexical decision should be undisturbed for words of all types (because it can be done on the basis of access to an entry in the orthographic input lexicon), but written word comprehension should be disturbed in a way that is characteristic of the central impairment in access to semantics; because this deficit is central, a qualitatively similar comprehension disturbance should be found with auditory word presentation, but word comprehension should be independent of factors, such as spelling-to-sound regularity, that affect the patient's ability to access phonology.

MK's performance precisely fits this third pattern of 'central surface dyslexia'. His visual lexical decision is very accurate with words of all types, including irregular words. Word comprehension does not depend on a word's spelling regularity, although his ability to pronounce it does. Written word comprehension does, however, depend on a word's imageability; he is better at understanding concrete words than abstract words, and the same abstractness effect is found in spoken word comprehension. Evidence from naming tasks suggests that there is only a mild degree of word finding difficulty, and this reflects a central problem in using semantic information in word retrieval rather than any impairment to the phonological output lexicon itself.

We can therefore conclude that MK has no 'direct route' available for word reading, and he is forced to be a surface dyslexic in oral word reading because of a breakdown in a semantically based reading routine at a central level.

The relationship between 'semantic errors in repetition' and 'surface dyslexia'

In chapter 12 we argued that the occurrence of semantic errors in repetition was a sufficient but not necessary condition for the symptomcomplex of 'deep dysgraphia'. In support of this view we demonstrated that MK and all the previously reported patients who make semantic errors in repetition are 'deep dysgraphic' in writing to spoken dictation.

In the introduction we noted that several, but not all, of the patients who made semantic errors in repetition were also 'surface dyslexic' in oral word reading (in other cases the relevant information on oral reading is not available); as we demonstrated, this is also true for MK. Is this coincidence, or is there a systematic relationship?

We argued that, in order to exhibit the symptomcomplex associated with 'semantic errors in repetition', a patient must be repeating via a

14. Coltheart and Funnell (1987) distinguish, on purely theoretical grounds, seven possible patterns of underlying impairment that could result in 'surface dyslexic' reading.

semantically based routine, in which the semantic system was defective, or the processes of access to the semantic system were disturbed. In discussing different subtypes of 'surface dyslexia', we argued that 'central surface dyslexia' will result when the (putative) direct nonsemantic lexical reading routine is abolished, and there is a central deficit in the semantic system, or in access to it. Both 'semantic errors in repetition' and 'central surface dyslexia' require a central semantic problem of just the same kind; surface dyslexia will always occur in patients who make semantic errors in repetition where (i) the 'sublexical reading routine' is reasonably intact (and so nonword reading is (relatively) good), and (ii) the 'direct lexical reading routine' is abolished.

In this view, then, 'semantic errors in repetition' and 'central surface dyslexia' will not invariably be associated with one another. On the other hand 'semantic errors in repetition' entail one of the two processing deficits needed to produce 'central surface dyslexia'. Each of these symptomcomplexes is caused by multiple information-processing deficits; to the extent that they hold one of their causes in common, the relationship between them is not accidental.

The right hemisphere and semantic errors in reading, repetition, and writing to dictation

When a patient makes semantic errors in reading, repetition, or writing to dictation with single words, a number of other characteristic features are found in the same task. These make up the symptomcomplexes of 'deep dyslexia', 'semantic errors in repetition', and 'deep dysgraphia'. As table 36 shows, there is a remarkable degree of similarity across all three symptomcomplexes. In each case there seems to be an implicational hierarchy: every patient who makes semantic errors in a task will show all the remaining features in performing that task.

MK shows all these features in repetition and writing to dictation. We have argued that the set of characteristics arise because MK is relying on a semantic routine that is defective in specific ways, affecting particularly the processing of abstract words, function words, and words with grammatical affixes.

In accounting for the same set of characteristic features in 'deep dyslexic' reading, Coltheart (1980c, 1983) and Saffran, Bogyo, Schwartz, and Marin (1980) have suggested that these features reflect processing by a right hemisphere reading system. This particular set of features arise simply because these are the (normal) properties of the right hemisphere reading system. In support of this conjecture Coltheart (1980c) reviews a wide range of studies involving lateralized presentation of stimuli to normal subjects and information from split brain patients and from other brain

Table 36
Common characteristics of the symptomcomplexes of 'deep dyslexia', 'deep dysgraphia', and 'semantic errors in repetition'

	Deep dyslexia	Deep dysgraphia	Semantic errors in repetition
Error types	Semantic errors	Semantic errors	Semantic errors
	Morphological errors	Morphological errors	Morphological errors**
	Visual errors	Visual/ortho-graphic errors	Phonological errors
	Function word substitutions	Function word substitutions	Function word substitutions**
Imageability effect	High > low	High > low	High > low
Part of speech effect*	'Content words' > 'function words'	'Content words' > 'function words'	'Content words' > 'function words'
Effect of morphological complexity	Monomorphemic > affixed	Monomorphemic > affixed	Monomorphemic > affixed
Performance with nonwords	Impossible	Impossible	Impossible

*The effect may only be found when imageability is not controlled between the lists
**Some of the patients described in section 1 do not appear to make these errors. It is unclear whether they were tested with the stimuli that are most likely to elicit the errors.

damaged subjects, and claims that the same set of features can be found in right hemisphere processing in these groups. Thus the right hemisphere reading system, Coltheart claims, is unable to process nonwords, has semantic information available only for concrete words, and is unable to process function words or suffixes.[15]

In this formulation, the coherence of the 'deep dyslexic' symptomcomplex reflects the characteristics of the right hemisphere reading system. If this is the case then, as Coltheart, Patterson, and Marshall (1987) note, the coherence of the symptomcomplexes of 'semantic errors in repetition' and 'deep dysgraphia' should also be attributed to the patients' reliance on a right hemisphere system for repetition or writing to dictation. So under the right hemisphere hypothesis we would need to claim that MK is repeating and writing with a right hemisphere system, but because his oral reading is not 'deep dyslexic', he is reading aloud with his left hemisphere. In the previous section we claimed that both MK's oral reading and his repetition reflected a central semantic breakdown; this involved the implicit assumption that he was using the same semantic system in reading as he was in

15. Patterson and Besner (1984) challenge Coltheart's interpretation of this evidence and argue that the reading of deep dyslexics differs in a number of ways from the characteristics of the right hemisphere lexical system.

repetition. The resemblance between the way semantic processes have broken down with visual and auditory presentation would in this account be entirely accidental. In understanding auditorily presented words, MK is better with concrete words than abstract ones because this is a feature of normal right hemisphere processing. In understanding visually presented words, he is better with concrete words than abstract ones because he is using a left hemisphere semantic system that happens to be damaged in a way that allows output resembling the output of the right hemisphere system.

The proposal that MK relies on two separate semantic systems for auditorily and visually presented words has a further problem. If there are separate semantic systems, MK should have great difficulty in tasks in which words have to be matched on the basis of meaning, when one word is presented visually and the other auditorily. Yet when we presented the 'Pyramids and Palm Trees' test in the form where MK had to match one spoken word to one of two written words, he managed 45/52—a quite respectable level of performance in view of his difficulties in spoken word comprehension. Clearly cross-modal semantic matching presents him with no particular difficulty.

A version of the right hemisphere hypothesis in which MK accesses separate semantic systems in each hemisphere for visually and auditorily presented words is therefore untenable. A second version would be that MK comprehends both spoken and written words with his right hemisphere, but that his output is from his left hemisphere, which also retains the routines needed for sublexical reading and sublexical copying. His spoken output in reading or repetition and written output to dictation result from transfer of postsemantic information from the right hemisphere to the left hemisphere output lexicons. This version of the right hemisphere hypothesis makes almost precisely the same predictions as the account we have offered above. It uses the same set of modules, having the same performance characteristics. It goes beyond our account in claiming that some components—the input lexicons and the cognitive system—are located in the right hemisphere and the others are located in the left hemisphere. Our account was not committed to any particular localization of the modules involved in the processing of words. To that extent it is equally compatible with this version of the right hemisphere hypothesis or the proposal that MK is relying exclusively on left hemisphere lexical processes.

The data from other patients reviewed in the introduction show multiple dissociations between different patients in whether they show these three symptomcomplexes (see Marshall 1977). Bub and Kertesz's (1982) patient JC shows 'deep dysgraphia' without either 'deep dyslexia' or 'semantic errors in repetition'. All of the patients who make 'semantic errors in repetition' are 'deep dysgraphic' but none are 'deep dyslexic'. All 'deep dyslexic' patients are also 'deep dysgraphic' (see Coltheart, Patterson, and Marshall 1987). Under a right hemisphere account we would have to claim that each of these sets of patients does some of these tasks with the right hemisphere and others with the left. We do not yet have a single account of a patient who shows 'deep dyslexia', 'deep dysgraphia', and 'semantic errors in repetition'. This patient would be one who relies on the right hemisphere for all three tasks. We might expect this to be a common feature of aphasic patients with large left hemisphere lesions. Under our alternative hypothesis, the occurrence of semantic errors in any task depends on three independent deficits. Semantic errors in reading will only co-occur with semantic errors in repetition when the 'direct routes' and the 'sublexical routines' are unavailable for both tasks, together with some lexical-semantic impairment. This particular collocation of functional lesions will only occur by chance, and we would therefore not often expect to identify patients with the triple symptomcomplex. The apparent rarity of patients of this kind provides weak evidence against a right hemisphere account of 'deep dyslexia', 'deep dysgraphia', and 'semantic errors in repetition'.

Chapter 14
On Single Subjects, Syndromes, and Symptoms

This book is a detailed account of some aspects of language performance in one aphasic subject, MK. It is one of many examples from the last ten years of studies devoted to individual brain damaged patients. There was an earlier era when neuropsychology dealt in detailed descriptions of single patients. Following the development of the Wernicke-Lichtheim model, many different aphasic cases were described in its terms. The purpose of the Wernicke-Lichtheim model was very similar to the purpose of the lexical model we have used:

> The theory of aphasia, here proposed, permits a consolidation of the diversified picture of the disorder. The diverse variety of symptoms which formerly had presented new riddles to each investigator does not now seem so striking, but may be predicted according to the laws of symptom-combination...Just as the analysis of the normal speech process on the basis of different centres permits one to incorporate the manifold forms of aphasia within a broader framework, so it allows an explanation of most of the contradictions which up to now had seemed so striking. (Wernicke 1874, p. 143 in 1977 translation)

Lichtheim saw the purpose of his model as presenting a position that could be falsified by data:

> I am well aware of the restricted foundations on which we may safely build, and what a space theoretical reasoning has still to occupy in the discussion. If I have, nevertheless, not kept my views to myself it was on the principle, that we must not recoil from the consequences deducible from our hypotheses. In proportion as we draw these conclusions, we shall obtain the necessary data whereby to correct, or if need be abandon, them. (Lichtheim 1885, p. 484)

Henry Head describes the excitement that he felt as young doctor in discovering that this schema could be used to make sense of the patterns of aphasic language. By 1926, however, he was disillusioned; he wrote that those operating within the schema were "compelled to lop and twist their cases to fit the procrustean bed of their hypothetical conceptions" (Head 1926, p. 53).

How, then, can our study avoid the twin problems of twisting the data from the patient to fit the theory or of *ad hoc* elaboration of the theory to fit the data from the patient?

Syndromes

Shallice (1979a) assembles arguments in favor of studying single patients; in particular he suggests that, in this way, neuropsychology can avoid the problem of averaging over qualitatively heterogeneous groups of patients. However, investigations of single patients confront the problem of replication. How can we be sure that a particular result is true, and therefore replicable? How can we be sure that our particular patient is not "in some way, premorbidly atypical" (p. 194)?

Shallice's answer is to identify the patient's syndrome. By this he means,

> a collection of symptoms that occur together because of the presence of a certain type of impairment to a certain type of functional subsystem or to particular subsystems - "pure" and "mixed" syndromes, respectively. Functional subsystems may be identified with information processing units [...] although it remains possible that any individual unit in a flow diagram may, in turn, be fractionated into more elementary functional subsystems.

Notice that, as Shallice points out, he is using the term 'syndrome' in a quite different way than it is usually used in neuropsychology. When authors talk, for example, of a 'parietal lobe syndrome' they mean a set of symptoms that occur together because they are all associated with damage to a particular area of the brain (see Marshall 1982); but as Benton (1961) demonstrated, the symptoms of the parietal lobe syndrome can all dissociate from from each other. The syndrome cannot therefore be attributed to a common *functional* cause. In this sense a syndrome is any set of symptoms that have a statistical tendency to occur together; they need do so only because they are caused by damage in anatomically related areas of the brain. Used in this way, the classical aphasia syndromes of the Wernicke-Lichtheim schema may have some use. Modern studies using methods of brain scanning have broadly confirmed that there is a statistical relationship between particular lesion sites and aphasic syndromes. However, this association is less than perfect at the level of individual patients. As Poeck, de Bleser, and Keyserlingk (1984) point out, there may be no area of the brain that is damaged in all of a set of patients who all have the same aphasic syndrome. And as Basso, Lecours, Moraschini, and Vanier (1985) show, there are exceptional patients with one variety of aphasic syndrome, where the lesion is in the area responsible for another syndrome. Therefore there is no necessary association between an aphasic syndrome and damage to a particular area of the brain.

In what Shallice describes as functional terms, this work with MK demonstrates that 'Wernicke's aphasia' cannot be called a syndrome. As the present definition stands, the label will be assigned to patients with a variety of different functional impairments.

To account for MK's processing of single words, we had to postulate eight different functional impairments. We could follow Shallice (1979) and call this a 'mixed syndrome'. We are skeptical whether there is any point in this: in the model of single word processing that we have used, there are (about) 27 components (boxes or arrows) that could plausibly be independently impaired. There will be $2^{27} - 1 = 134,217,727$ different possible combinations of impairments (Marshall 1984). Of these just 27 will be 'pure' syndromes; there will be $27!/(19! \times 8!) = 2,220,075$ different mixed syndromes that have eight different impairments. So we assume that other patients with the same qualitative pattern of impairment as MK will probably be rare; we see no purpose in claiming to have 'discovered' a new syndrome. As most aphasic patients will show multiple impairments (and therefore in Shallice's terms 'mixed syndromes'), assigning them syndrome labels is not a productive strategy.

In the present context, to abandon the notion of syndrome does not seem particularly surprising; many authors have argued for just such a change (e.g., Caramazza 1984; Coltheart 1985; Ellis 1987; Howard 1985b; Marshall 1982, 1986; Schwartz 1984). But Shallice makes one specific claim for the utility of the syndrome concept:

> Without such a concept, treacherous though it is to apply, there would be no useful meaning to the idea of replication of findings on any other patient. Results then, might have considerable curiosity value, but would not be part of a scientific data base.   (p. 189)

The next section is a defense of our data from MK. We will argue that it is of more than curiosity value and is open to scientific replication. Our data and arguments are truly part of a scientific data base.

Replication

It seems unlikely that we will find another patient with quite the same pattern of impairments as MK. In what sense then can we claim that our findings with him are replicable and have some real validity?

We have tried to ensure this replicability in a number of ways. First we have used *internal replication*. In almost every case we have tested for a particular effect with MK on two different occasions. Wherever possible we have tried to test one particular function (or variable) with two different stimulus sets, and in different sessions. On other occasions we have simply had to repeat testing. Apart from repeated testing, we have replicated by comparisons across tasks and across methods of analysis. Thus, for example, we found no effect of word frequency on word repetition using balanced sets of items. We replicated this in our analysis of repetition responses to a large corpus. We extended the way in which we replicated by comparisons across modalities and tasks. Thus, for example, we showed that the factors affecting writing to dictation were almost identical to the factors affecting oral word repetition. But there was an exception; while repetition was better for longer words than shorter ones, writing to dictation was unaffected by word length. First we replicated this difference in the analysis of a larger corpus. We then hypothesized that the difference was due to a problem in correct written production of longer words; this same problem should therefore be evident in other tasks involving written output. We were able to support this hypothesis in both written naming and delayed copying. Thus there are two senses in which we have been able to use internal replication; first, in repeating results with different stimulus materials, in different sessions, or with different procedures. Second, we were able to show that performance in other kinds of tasks was consistent with the kinds of underlying impairment that the first kinds of tests had indicated. In these ways we have ensured that our results with MK are not chance results and do not depend on a few selected observations. By using this kind of specific and comprehensive testing, we are able to have real confidence in our results.

Internal replication allows us to show that, even if no other identical patient is ever found, we have a true picture of MK's performance. Even if an identical patient is not found, there is a sense in which we can fruitfully compare across different patients. We described MK as showing a number of different symptomcomplexes. We chose this term instead of syndrome deliberately.[16] Shallice used the term 'syndrome' to refer to a set of symptoms caused by a defined set of one or more underlying functional impairments. We have used 'symptomcomplex' to refer to a set of symptoms reflecting the operation of a particular functional system, without wishing to delimit the impairments that might underlie the complex. Thus, we have suggested that the term 'surface dyslexia' should be used to apply to patients who in reading aloud are (i) more accurate with words whose spelling reflects a consistent relationship between spelling and sound than those where the relationship is exceptional, and (ii) make phonologically

16. We are aware that many authors from Wernicke (1874) to Marshall (1982) have used 'symptomcomplex' as a synonym of syndrome. We want to use these terms in two distinct ways.

plausible errors in reading (Howard and Franklin 1987, and the present work). We did this because these two features reflect reliance on a sublexical routine in reading aloud. We argued that this must reflect a breakdown in lexical routines for retrieving the spoken forms corresponding to written words. As we showed earlier, there are case histories of 'surface dyslexic' patients that allow us to distinguish three distinct levels of impairment to lexical reading processes, and on theoretical grounds Coltheart and Funnell (1987) suggest at least seven possible causes. Thus the functional impairments will not necessarily be the same across a set of 'surface dyslexics'; thus it cannot be called a syndrome. But the two symptoms we have advanced as the symptomcoplex hold together because they reflect reliance on a sublexical reading procedure. In a similar vein we have argued that the symptomcomplex accompanying semantic errors in repetition reflects the use of a lexical-semantic routine for word repetition, even though a number of qualitatively functional impairments might cause the symptomcomplex. Thus one way in which we have assessed whether MK's impairments reflect some idiosyncratic form of cortical organization is by comparing him with other patients who show the same, or related, symptomcomplexes. Thus, for example, we were concerned to show that his pattern of performance in repetition was consistent with what we can deduce from descriptions of other patients who have similar symptomcomplexes. Seen in these terms, almost none of the individual features in MK's performance are unique; to this extent they all find replication in the literature. In order to facilitate future comparisons across patients, we have tried to use with MK tests that have been published or are widely used. We have used these lists even where it happens that they do not control some essential variable. This is so that future researchers can use the same tests with their patients and assess the extent to which there is quantitative and qualitative similarity with MK by comparing the results. Thus we can increase confidence in our results by showing that they are consistent with other findings in the literature.

There is a third and even more abstract way in which we can demonstrate the reliability of our findings with MK: by showing that our findings are interpretable within a theoretical framework that depends upon and is able to incorporate results from other aphasic patients and from laboratory experiments with normal subjects. Coltheart (1984) argues that, in making generalizations across patients,

> The generalisations do not take the form of claiming that there exists a single syndrome which many patients exhibit. Instead these generalisations take the form of claiming that there exists a single model of the relevant cognitive system which can offer interpretations of the various sets of symptoms exhibited by various different patients.   (p. 6)

Thus we have devoted part of chapter 12 of this book to examining the ways in which data from MK converge with data and theoretical positions that draw their motivation from the traditional source for cognitive psychology—laboratory experiments with normal subjects. We showed, for instance, that the way that MK uses contextual information in auditory word recognition is compatible with a variety of theories, such as Marslen-Wilson's 'cohort model' or McLelland and Elman's 'TRACE', that suppose that it is interaction between bottom-up sensory information and top-down contextual information that drives word recognition. On the issue of whether there are separate phonological lexicons for input an output, we showed that our results with MK reinforce the other experimental evidence from priming studies (Monsell 1987) and dual tasks (Shallice et al. 1985) with normal subjects, that together point toward separate lexical systems.

Taken together, these lines of evidence suggest that, even though no patient quite like MK has ever been described before, our findings with him are reliable. We have shown the internal consistency of his results; we have shown consistency between his performance and other patients with related symptomcomplexes; and we have shown that these results can have an economical and theoretically revealing interpretation in terms of lexical models able to account for both neuropsychological data and laboratory results with normal people. We hope that we have established that an in-depth study of a single aphasic patient can be worthwhile and scientifically revealing.

Postscript

We have provided in this book an exhaustive analysis of MK's performance in a wide range of tasks involving processing of single words. Some readers may feel that this type of analysis is too mechanistic because so many factors have been deliberately excluded from the analysis. It leaves out all the aspects of language use and of how language is an integral part of (most) social relationships. It leaves out issues of the control of language processes, of intentions, wishes, and desires. It leaves out using language for conversation, for argument, and for loving. And, most fundamentally, we have excluded all consideration of the consequences for MK, and for his family and friends, of his being aphasic. We have avoided any consideration of how this has changed the relationships that MK can have and the frustrations and limitations it imposes on his life.

Although we have not considered these issues, we still think that they are important. We are both aphasia therapists, and one of our aims in interacting with MK was to try to 'improve' his language, to try to lessen the limitations that his aphasia has imposed on his life. Over the years that we have been seeing him, we have tried a number of different treatment approaches, partly in order to improve his language but also as an experimental tool in trying to understand his problems (see Howard and Patterson 1988). None have been conspicuously successful, and so no results seem worth reporting. We wonder, sometimes, whether our failures in therapy are the inevitable result of multiple and severe processing impairments. The difficulty that is the greatest impediment to communication is probably his severe problem in sentence comprehension, which we document elsewhere (Howard and Franklin 1988). There seems to be no 'alternative' strategy that MK can use to circumvent a problem of such magnitude (see Beauvois and Derouesne 1982).

We are constantly aware that MK's aphasia is a very major handicap; communication is difficult. Much of his work with his therapists is hard for him, both emotionally and cognitively. One day he brought in a piece that he had written about his stroke. We think it is best described as a poem; it conveys very effectively the pain and difficulty of his aphasia. We reproduce it here with the original spelling and the original format:

Stroke

Therapy Dully, <u>Brain</u> (-SWIVEL!!), helps?, storm,
(no blind), cells, dotty, dizzy, silly,
Mental, walls-lorries?, loonies
Sensible, drilled,
Strings, <u>wooly</u>, cracked,
Splinters, swivels, rotate, move
Speckled, eyes blockage, cleared,
Slender, blobs, bulbs, lump,
Red Pills, pneumatic, trauma,
ragged, scribble, zigzag, flapping-flips,
(water wings?), feet-cold, box-voices,
Numbs, jumble, game-lame,
Peg-wooden-balls—stockets—toes not-got,
Springs-terror-tears <u>bounce</u>, cracks,
honeycombs, chord, grids (like lattice),
talks, carbuncle, films-brain,
blurred, GENTLE-comprehension,   ROCKET!!!

Sharp, corners, edge.
Fog, Shutter, shadows, opaque,
bulks-heavy,
Twang, chords, cords, tendons
bulk-bloody
Garble (talking?)
baloons, double-eye,
Noise, chatty, speech
Vocal, head, cranium, <u>mentally</u>
double-visions.

Therapy—speech, handicap,
Stammer, wire? screws,
Stammer,
Ejaculation,
ragged,
splint,
creaks,

Cloud-wooly physical
Chiropodist, babble
(gloom—not very well!)
Quiet, try good-boy,

Concertains, grids, <u>pains</u> sometimes
—with head!! Blood
try for an puncture,
Rubbery,

Muscular
Weakness

Appendix 1
Matching Data for Word Sets

Table A
Matching data for imageability matched content and function word lists

	Content words	Function words
Number of items	60	40
Number of letters		
range	3−7	3−7
mean	4.82	4.32
sd	1.13	1.19
Log Kucera and Francis word frequency		
range	2.0−3.3	2.1−4.5
mean	2.41	3.01
sd	0.29	0.50
Imageability		
range	271−350	271−346
mean	312	308
sd	23	23

Table B
Matching data for frequency matched content and function word lists

	Content words	Function words
Number of items	50	50
Number of letters		
range	2–7	2–7
mean	4.48	4.48
sd	1.14	1.14
Log Kucera and Francis word frequency		
range	2.0–3.2	2.0–3.2
mean	2.68	2.68
sd	0.28	0.28
Log Thorndike and Lorge word frequency		
range	2.6–4.0	2.8–3.9
mean	3.35	3.34
sd	0.38	0.32
Imageability		
range	263–632	206–428
mean	445	297
sd	99	62

Only 45 of the content words and 38 of the function words have imageability values in the MRC database; the imageability data are based on these subsets.

Table C
Matching data for one- two- and three-syllable word lists

	One-syllable words	Two-syllable words	Three-syllable words
Number of items	30	30	30
Number of letters			
range	4–6	5–9	6–10
mean	4.73	7.07	8.07
sd	.68	1.00	1.03
Number of phonemes			
range	3–5	4–7	6–8
mean	3.67	5.53	7.03
sd	.66	.90	.67
Log Kucera and Francis word frequency*			
range	−.3–2.1	−.3–2.1	−.3–2.0
mean	0.89	0.88	0.87
sd	0.71	0.72	0.73
Imageability			
range	506–637	505–642	505–655
mean	603	603	603
sd	36	36	37

*Where a word did not appear in the Kucera and Francis word count, we arbitrarily assigned it a frequency of 0.5 wpm for the purpose of calculating log word frequencies.

Table D
Matching data for high and low imageability and high and low frequency word lists

	High imageability, low frequency	High imageability, high frequency	Low imageability, low frequency	Low imageability, high frequency
Number of items	20	20	20	20
Number of letters				
range	4–6	4–6	4–6	4–6
mean	4.75	4.75	4.75	4.75
sd	.85	.85	.85	.85
Number of phonemes				
range	3–6	2–5	1–6	2–5
mean	3.60	3.60	3.85	3.50
sd	.82	.94	1.04	.89
Log Kucera and Francis word frequency				
range	.78–1.28	2.00–2.30	.70–1.28	2.01–2.30
mean	1.09	2.15	1.05	2.17
sd	0.13	0.10	0.16	0.08
Imageability				
range	572–637	575–634	315–397	315–396
mean	602	601	364	364
sd	20	20	30	31

Table E
Matching data for regular and irregular word lists of high and low imageability

	High imageability, regular	High imageability, irregular	Low imageability, regular	Low imageability, irregular
Number of items	65	65	55	55
Number of letters				
range	3−6	3−6	3−6	3−6
mean	4.46	4.48	4.60	4.60
sd	.73	.73	.81	.81
Number of phonemes				
range	2−5	1−5	2−6	1−6
mean	3.57	3.51	3.75	3.67
sd	.73	.92	1.08	.96
Log Kucera and Francis word frequency				
range	0.30−2.63	0.30−2.67	0.0−2.79	0.0−2.63
mean	1.37	1.38	1.38	1.37
sd	0.62	0.62	0.76	0.78
Imageability				
range	507−636	518−647	222−394	210−398
mean	584	585	337	340
sd	32	33	44	44

Table F
Matching data for matched high and low imageability lists

	High imageability words	Low imageability words
Number of items	100	100
Number of letters		
range	4−7	4−7
mean	5.20	5.20
sd	0.98	0.98
Log Kucera and Francis word frequency		
range	1.30−2.32	1.30−2.34
mean	1.72	1.72
sd	0.28	0.28
Imageability		
range	553−646	300−399
mean	599	361
sd	21	29

Appendix 2
MK's Spoken Description of the Story of Cinderella

"So I want me to talk about, you want me to talk about er er princess, well, she's not princess yet but she does eventually. It was Cinderella and she had a, she had a, she had a about a, she had an old or ugly, an old, two old sisters. And she came up to find out for herself. Er what did she do? She had to do dirty and she had to do work all the time up the kitchens and round. And um that little bit sometime that she got a little bit of a little bit of hungry, not very many though, and she got clean after a while and then she wanted to go out, then she wanted to get out to, to see, to see, to see herself, to get some um um

"I think I've got to talk this bit slowly. I'm so sorry. I forget what these things are. She, she wanted to start, get something to, er, she wanted to do a dress for herself, er and then eventually, she had to [unintelligible]. She get a nice places for her.

"I think I'll, I'm going to take it a little bit time, because I'm always slow to start in the morning. But by, in about, about a, in about a few minutes I hope it'll get much better. But at the moment I don't know too much just now. Um but now I then have to talk with then. I remember finding a, a, had to get a thing called a pumpkin. She got one, then she went out with a, a young, a young prince wanted to get hold of her. And she took, the man took Cinderella outside to get something to eat for herself too-very good one. She didn't have a drink but she liked it all the same. Um er but um but she didn't like the, that other the old two ugly, ugly women. She didn't like them at all very much. Um and 'cause they wanted themselves to get out and they wanted to get, er get shoes.

"For, for herself she, the two women wanted to have good shoes. But Cinderella wanted to have a nice little one slipper. A small one, I remember that one. And eventually she put the slipper upon herself, and then she pick it up and um everyone said it's perfectly all right for you. And it became, it came up by um /dəˈsɪlvə/ as well as slipper as well. And then she went across to the pumpkins, all, all down, she went down across back to her home and listened to herself. Is there anything else to specially about these things? Sorry."

References

Albert, M. L., Goodglass, H., Helm, N. A., Rubens, A. B., and Alexander, M. P. (1981). *Clinical aspects of dysphasia*. Vienna: Springer Verlag.

Allport, D. A. (1983). Language and cognition. In R. Harris (ed.), *Approaches to language*. Oxford: Pergamon.

Allport, D. A. (1984a). Speech production and comprehension: one lexicon or two? In W. Prinz and A. F. Sanders (eds.), *Cognition and motor processes*. Berlin: Springer Verlag.

Allport, D. A. (1984b). Auditory-verbal short-term memory and conduction aphasia. In H. Bouma and D. G. Bouwhuis (eds.), *Attention and performance X; control of language processes*. Hillsdale, New Jersey: Lawrence Erlbaum.

Allport, D. A. (1985). Distributed memory, modular sub-systems and dysphasia. In S. K. Newman and R. Epstein (eds.) *Current perspectives in dysphasia*. Edinburgh: Churchill Livingstone.

Allport, D. A., and Funnell, E. (1981). Components of the mental lexicon. *Philosophical Transactions of the Royal Society of London*, B295, 397−410.

Aronoff, M. (1976) *Word formation in generative grammar*. Cambridge, Massachusetts: MIT Press.

Auerbach, S. H., Allard, A., Naeser, M., Alexander, M. P., and Albert, M. L. (1982). Pure word deafness: analysis of a case with bilateral lesions and a defect at the prephonemic level. *Brain*, 105, 271−300.

Baddeley, A. D. (1986). *Working memory*. Oxford: Oxford University Press.

Baker, E., Blumstein, S. E., and Goodglass, H. (1981). Interaction between phonological and semantic factors in auditory comprehension. *Neuropsychologia*, 19, 1−15.

Basso, A., Lecours, A. R., Moraschini, S., and Vanier, M. (1985). Anatomoclinical correlations of the aphasias as defined through computerised tomography: exceptions. *Brain and Language*, 26, 201−229.

Bauer, D. W., and Stanovich, K. E. (1980). Lexical access and the spelling-to-sound regularity effect. *Memory & Cognition* 8, 424−432.

Beauvois, M-F. (1982). Optic aphasia; a process of interaction between vision and language. *Philosophical Transactions of the Royal Society of London*, B298, 35−48.

Beauvois, M-F. and Derouesné, J. (1982). Recherche en neuropsychologie et rééducation; quels rapports? In X. Seron and C. Laterre (eds.), *Rééduquer le cerveau*. Brussels: Mardaga.

Benton, A. L. (1961). The fiction of the 'Gerstmann syndrome'. *Journal of Neurology, Neurosurgery and Psychiatry*, 24, 176−181.

Bishop, D. V. M., and Byng, S. (1984). Assessing semantic comprehension: methodological considerations and a new clinical test. *Cognitive Neuropsychology*, 1, 233−244.

Blank, M. J., and Foss, D. J. (1978). Semantic facilitation and lexical access during sentence processing. *Memory and Cognition*, 6, 644−652.

Blumstein, S. E., Baker, E., and Goodglass, H. (1977). Phonological factors in auditory comprehension in aphasia. *Neuropsychologia*, 15, 19−30.

Bonvincini, G. (1905). Ueber subcorticale sensorische Aphasie. *Jahrbuch für Psychiatrie und Neurologie*, 26, 126−299.

Borod, J. C., Goodglass, H., and Kaplan, E. (1980). Normative data on the Boston Diagnostic Aphasia Examination, parietal lobe battery, and the Boston Naming Test. *Journal of Clinical Neuropsychology*, 2, 209−215.

Bramwell, B. (1897). Illustrative cases of aphasia (case 11). *Lancet*, 1, 1256−1259. Reprinted with an introduction by A. W. Ellis, 1984, in *Cognitive Neuropsychology*, 1, 245−258.

Bub, D., and Kertesz, A. (1982). Deep agraphia. *Brain and Language*, 17, 146−165.

Bub, D., Cancelliere, A., and Kertesz, A. (1985). Whole word and analytic translation of spelling to sound in a non-semantic reader. In K. E. Patterson, J. C. Marshall, and M. Coltheart (eds.), *Surface dyslexia: neuropsychological and cognitive analyses of phonological reading*. London: Lawrence Erlbaum.

Butterworth, B. L. (1979). Hesitation and the production of verbal paraphasias and neologisms in jargon aphasia. *Brain and Language*, 8, 133−161.

Butterworth, B. L. (1980). Some constraints on models of language production. In B. L. Butterworth (ed.), *Language production, volume 1: speech and talk*. London: Academic Press.

Butterworth, B. L. (1988). Lexical access in speech production. In W. Marslen-Wilson (ed.), *Lexical representation and process*. London: MIT press.

Butteworth, B. L., and Howard, D. (1987). Paragrammatisms. *Cognition*, 26, 1−37.

Butterworth, B. L., Howard, D., and McLoughlin, P. J. (1984). The semantic deficit in aphasia: the relationship between semantic errors in auditory comprehension and picture naming. *Neuropsychologia*, 22, 409−426.

Byng, S., Coltheart, M., Masterson, J., Prior, M., and Riddoch, J. (1984). Bilingual biscriptal deep dyslexia. *Quarterly Journal of Experimental Psychology*, 36A, 417−433.

Caplan, D., Vanier, M., and Baker, C. (1986). A case study of reproduction conduction aphasia I; word production. *Cognitive Neuropsychology*, 3, 99−128.

Caramazza, A. (1984) The logic of neuropsychological research and the problem of patient classification in aphasia. *Brain and Language*, 21, 9−20.

Caramazza, A., Berndt, R., and Basili, A. (1983). The selective impairment of phonological processing; a case study. *Brain and Language*, 18, 128−174.

Caramazza, A., Miceli, G., and Villa, G. (1986). The role of the (output) phonological buffer in reading, writing and repetition. *Cognitive Neuropsychology*, 3, 37−76.

Caramazza, A., Miceli, G., Villa, G., and Romani, C. (1987). The role of the graphemic buffer in spelling. *Cognition*, 26, 59−85.

Clarke, R., and Morton, J. (1983). Cross-modality facilitation in tachistoscopic word recognition. *Quarterly Journal of Experimental Psychology*, 35A, 79−96.

Coltheart, M. (1978). Lexical access in simple reading tasks. In G. Underwood (ed.), *Strategies of information processing*. London: Academic Press.

Coltheart, M. (1980a). Analysing acquired disorders of reading. Unpublished manuscript, Birkbeck College, London.

Coltheart, M. (1980b). The semantic error: types and theories. In M. Coltheart, K. E. Patterson, and J. C. Marshall (eds.), *Deep dyslexia*. London: Routledge & Kegan Paul.

Coltheart, M. (1980c). Deep dyslexia: a right hemisphere hypothesis. In M. Coltheart, K. E. Patterson and J. C. Marshall, (eds.) *Deep dyslexia*. London: Routledge & Kegan Paul.

Coltheart, M. (1981). The MRC Psycholinguistic Database. *Quarterly Journal of Experimental Psychology*, 33A, 497−505.

Coltheart, M. (1983) The right hemisphere and disorders of reading. In A. Young (ed.), *Functions of the right hemisphere*. London: Academic Press.

Coltheart, M. (1984). Editorial, *Cognitive Neuropsychology*, 1, 1−8.

Coltheart, M. (1985). Cognitive neuropsychology and the study of reading. In M. I. Posner and O. S. M. Marin (eds.), *Attention and performance, XI*. Hillsdale, New Jersey: Lawrence Erlbaum.

Coltheart, M., and Funnell, E. (1987). Reading and writing: one lexicon or two? In D. A. Allport, D. MacKay, W. Prinz, and E. Scheerer (eds.), *Language perception and production; common processes in listening, speaking, reading and writing*. London: Academic Press.

Coltheart, M., Besner, D., Jonasson, J. T., and Davelaar, E. (1979). Phonological encoding in the lexical decision task. *Quarterly Journal of Experimental Psychology*, 31, 489−507.

Coltheart, M., Masterson, J., Byng, S., Prior, M., and Riddoch, J. (1983). Surface dyslexia. *Quarterly Journal of Experimental Psychology*, 35A, 469−496.

Coltheart, M., Patterson, K. E., and Marshall, J. C. (1980). *Deep dyslexia*. London: Routledge & Kegan Paul.

Coltheart, M., Patterson, K. E., and Marshall, J. C. (1987). Deep dyslexia since 1980. In M. Coltheart, K. E. Patterson, and J. C. Marshall (eds.) *Deep dyslexia*. London: Routledge & Kegan Paul, second edition.

Coltheart, M., Sartori, G., and Job, R. (eds.) (1987). *The cognitive neuropsychology of language*. London: Lawrence Erlbaum Associates.

Davis, A. (1987). Semantic deficits and their relationship to naming disorders in head injured patients. Unpublished MSc thesis, City University, London.

Deloche, G., Andreewsky, E., and Desi, M. (1982). Surface dyslexia: a case report and some theoretical implications to reading models. *Brain and Language*, 15, 12−31.

Derouesné, J., and Beauvois, M-F. (1985). The "phonemic" stage in the non-lexical reading process: evidence from a case of phonological alexia. In K. E. Patterson, J. C. Marshall, and M. Coltheart (eds.), *Surface dyslexia: neuropsychological and cognitive analyses of phonological reading*. London: Lawrence Erlbaum.

Dodd, B., and Campbell, R. (eds.) (1987). *Hearing by eye*. London: Lawrence Erlbaum Associates.

Duhamel, J-R., and Poncet, M. (1986). Deep dysphasia in a case of phonemic deafness: role of the right hemisphere in auditory language comprehension. *Neuropsychologia*, 24, 769−799.

Dunn, A. (1965). *The Peabody Picture Vocabulary Test*. Minneapolis: American Guidance Service.

Ellis, A. W. (1982). Spelling and writing (and reading and speaking). In A. W. Ellis (ed.), *Normality and pathology in cognitive function*. London: Academic Press.

Ellis, A. W. (1987). Intimations of modularity or the modelarity of mind: doing cognitive neuropsychology without syndromes. In M. Coltheart, G. Sartori, and R. Job (eds.), *The cognitive neuropsychology of language*. London: Lawrence Erlbaum Associates.

Ellis, A. W., and Marshall, J. C. (1977). Semantic errors or statistical flukes? A note on Allport's 'On knowing the meaning of words we are unable to report'. *Quarterly Journal of Experimental Psychology*, 30, 569−575.

Forster, K. I., and Chambers, S. M. (1973). Lexical access and naming time. *Journal of Verbal Learning and Verbal Behaviour*, 12, 627−635.

Funnell, E. (1983a). Phonological processes in reading: new evidence from acquired dyslexia. *British Journal of Psychology*, 74, 159−180.

Funnell, E. (1983b). Ideographic communication and word class differences in aphasia. Unpublished PhD thesis, University of Reading.

Funnell, E., and Allport, D. A. (1987). Non-linguistic cognition and word meanings: neuropsychological exploration of common mechanisms. In D. A. Allport, D. MacKay, W. Prinz, and E. Scheerer (eds.), *Language perception and production; common processes in listening, speaking, reading and writing*. London: Academic Press.

Franklin, S. (1989). Dissociations in auditory word comprehension; evidence from nine 'fluent' aphasic patients. *Aphasiology*, in press.

Gainotti, G., Caltagirone, C., and Ibba, A. (1975). Semantic and phonemic aspects of auditory comprehension in aphasia. *Linguistics*, 154/155, 15−29.

Garrett, M. F. (1980). Levels of processing in sentence production. In B. L. Butterworth (ed.), *Language production, volume 1; speech and talk*. London: Academic Press.

Glushko, R. J. (1979). The organisation and activation of orthographic knowledge in reading aloud. *Journal of Experimental Psychology: Human Perception and Performance*, 5, 674−691.

Goldblum, M-C. (1979). Auditory analogue of deep dyslexia. *Experimental Brain Research*, Supplement II: hearing and speech, 397−405.

Goldblum, M-C. (1980). Un équivalent de la dyslexie profonde dans la modalité auditive. *Grammatica*, 7, 157−177.

Goldblum, M-C. (1985). Word comprehension in surface dyslexia. In K. E. Patterson, J. C. Marshall, and M. Coltheart (eds.), *Surface dyslexia: neuropsychological and cognitive analyses of phonological reading* . London: Lawrence Erlbaum.

Goldstein, K. (1906). Ein beitrag zur Lehre von der Aphasie. *Journal für Psychologie und Neurologie*, 7, 172−188.

Goldstein, K. (1948). *Language and language disturbances*. New York: Grune and Stratton.

Goldstein, M. N. (1974). Auditory agnosia for speech ("pure word deafness"). *Brain and Language*, 1, 195−204.

Goodglass, H., and Geschwind, N. (1976). Language disorders (aphasia). In E. C. Carterette and M. P. Friedman (eds.), *Handbook of perception, volume 7*. New York: Academic Press.

Goodglass, H., and Kaplan, E. (1972). *Assessment of aphasia and related disorders*. Philadelphia: Lea & Febiger.

Grosjean, F. (1980). Spoken word recognition processes and the gating paradigm. *Perception and Psychophysics*, 28, 267−283.

Hatfield, F. M. (1982). Diverses formes de disentégration du langage écrit et implications pour la ré-éducation. In X. Seron and C. Laterre (eds.), *Ré-éduquer le cerveau: logopédie, psychologie, neurologie*. Brussels: Pierre Mardaga.

Hatfield, F. M. (1983). Aspects of acquired dysgraphia and implications for reeducation. In C. Code and D. J. Muller (eds.), *Aphasia therapy*. London: Edward Arnold.

Hatfield, F. M. (1985). Visual and phonological factors in acquired dysgraphia. *Neuropsychologia*, 23, 13−29.

Hatfield, F. M., and Patterson, K. E. (1983). Phonological spelling. *Quarterly Journal of Exprimental Psychology*, 35A, 451−468.

Hatfield, F. M., and Patterson, K. E. (1984). Interpretation of spelling disorders in aphasia: impact of recent developments in cognitive psychology. In F. C. Rose (ed.), *Advances in neurology 42; progress in aphasiology*. New York: Raven.

Hécaen, H. (1972). *Introduction à la neuropsychologie*. Paris: Larousse.

Heilman, K. M., Rothi, L., Campanella, D., and Wolfson, S. (1979). Wernicke's and global aphasia without alexia. *Archives of Neurology*, 36, 129−133.

Henderson, L. (1985). Issues in the modelling of pronunciation assembly in normal reading. In, K. E. Patterson, J. C. Marshall, and M. Coltheart (eds.), *Surface dyslexia: neuropsychological and cognitive analyses of phonological reading*. London: Lawrence Erlbaum.

Henneberg, R. (1906). Ueber unvollstaendige reine Worttaubheit. *Monatsschrift für Psychiatrie und Neurologie*, 19, 17−38, 159−179.

Hier, D. B., and Mohr, J. P. (1977). Incongruous oral and written naming; evidence for a subdivision of the syndrome of Wernicke's aphasia. *Brain and Language*, 4, 115−126.

Hotopf, N. (1980) Slips of the pen. In U. Frith (ed.), *Cognitive processes in spelling*. London: Academic Press.

Howard, D. (1985a). The semantic organisation of the lexicon; evidence from aphasia. Unpublished PhD thesis, University of London.

Howard, D. (1985b). Agrammatism. In S. K. Newman and R. Epstein (eds.), *Current perspectives in dysphasia*. Edinburgh: Churchill Livingstone.

Howard, D. (1987). Reading without letters? In M. Coltheart, R. Job, and G. Sartori (eds.), *The cognitive neuropsychology of language*. London: Lawrence Erlbaum.

Howard, D., and Franklin, S. (1987). Three ways for understanding written words and their use in two contrasting cases of surface dyslexia. In D. A. Allport, D. MacKay, W. Prinz, and E. Scheerer (eds.), *Language perception and production; common processes in listening, speaking, reading and writing*. London: Academic Press.

Howard, D., and Franklin, S. (1988). Memory without rehearsal. In T. Shallice and G. Vallar (eds.), *The neurological impairment of short term memory*. Cambridge: Cambridge University Press.

Howard, D., and Orchard-Lisle, V. M. (1984). On the origin of semantic errors in naming; evidence from the case of a global aphasic. *Cognitive Neuropsychology*, 1, 163–190.

Howard, D., and Patterson, K. E. (unpublished). *The pyramids and palm trees test*.

Howard, D., and Patterson, K. E. (1988). Models for therapy. In X. Seron and G. Deloche (eds.), *Cognitive neuropsychological approaches to rehabilitation*. Hillsdale, New Jersey: Lawrence Erlbaum Associates.

Howard, D., Patterson, K. E., Franklin, S., Orchard-Lisle, V. M., and Morton, J. (1985). The facilitation of picture naming in aphasia. *Cognitive Neuropsychology*, 2, 41–80.

Humphreys, G. W., and Evett, L. J. (1985). Are there independent lexical and non-lexical routes in word processing? An evaluation of the dual-route theory of reading. *Behavioural and Brain Sciences*, 8, 689–740.

Kaplan, E., Goodglass, H., and Weintraub, S. (1976). *The Boston Naming Test*. Boston: Veteran's Administration.

Kay, J. (1985) Mechanisms of oral reading: a critical appraisal of cognitive models. In A. W. Ellis (ed.), *Progress in the psychology of language, volume 2*. London: Lawrence Erlbaum Associates.

Kay, J., and Lesser, R. (1985). The nature of phonological processing in oral reading: evidence from surface dyslexia. *Quarterly Journal of Experimental Psychology*, 37A, 39–81.

Kay, J., and Marcel, A. J. (1981). One process not two in reading aloud; lexical analogies do the work of non-lexical rules. *Quarterly Journal of Experimental Psychology*, 33A, 397–413.

Kay, J., and Patterson, K. E. (1985). Routes to meaning in surface dyslexia. In, K. E. Patterson, J. C. Marshall, and M. Coltheart (eds.), *Surface dyslexia: neuropsychological and cognitive analyses of phonological reading*. London: Lawrence Erlbaum.

Kempen, G., and Huijbers, P. (1983). The lexicalisation process in sentence production and naming: indirect selection of words. *Cognition*, 14, 185–209.

Klein, R., and Harper, J. (1956). The problem of agnosia in the light of a case of pure word deafness. *Journal of Mental Science*, 102, 112–120.

Kohn, S. E., and Friedman, R. B. (1986). Word meaning deafness: a phonological-semantic dissociation. *Cognitive Neuropsychology*, 3, 291–308.

Kremin, H. (1980). Deux stratégies de lecture dissociables par la pathologie: description d'un cas de dyslexie profonde et d'un cas de dyslexie de surface. *Grammatica*, 7, 131–156.

Kremin, H. (1985). Routes and strategies in surface dyslexia and dysgraphia. In, K. E. Patterson, J. C. Marshall, and M. Coltheart (eds.), *Surface dyslexia: neuropsychological and cognitive analyses of phonological reading*. London: Lawrence Erlbaum.

Kremin, H. (1986). Spared naming without comprehension. *Journal of Neurolinguistics*, 2, 131–150.

Kucera, H., and Francis, W. N. (1967). *A computational analysis of present-day American English*. Providence, Rhode Island: Brown University Press.

Levelt, W. J. M., and Maassen, B. (1981). Lexical search and order of mention in sentence production. In W. Klein and W. J. M. Levelt (eds.), *Crossing the boundaries in linguistics*. Dordrecht: Riedel.

Lichtheim, L. (1885). Ueber Aphasie. *Deutsches Archiv für klinische Medizin*, 36, 204–268. English translation, On aphasia, 1885. *Brain*, 7, 433–485.

Luria, A. R. (1947). *Travmaticheskaya afazia*. Moscow; Izd Akad Ped Nauk RSFSR. Translated by D. Bowden, 1970, as *Traumatic aphasia*. The Hague: Mouton.

Marcel, A. J. (1980). Surface dyslexia and beginning reading: a revised hypothesis of the pronunciation of print and its impairments. In M. Coltheart, K. E. Patterson, and J. C. Marshall (eds.), *Deep dyslexia*. London: Routledge & Kegan Paul.

Margolin, D. I., Marcel, A. J., and Carlson, N. R. (1985). Common mechanisms in dysnomia and post-semantic surface dyslexia: processing deficits and selective attention. In K. E. Patterson, J. C. Marshall, and M. Coltheart (eds.), *Surface dyslexia: neuropsychological and cognitive analyses of phonological reading*. London: Lawrence Erlbaum.

Marshall, J. C. (1976). Neuropsychological aspects of orthographic representation. In R. J. Wales and E. Walker (eds.), *New approaches to language mechanisms*. Amsterdam: North-Holland.

Marshall, J. C. (1982) What is a symptomcomplex? In M. A. Arbib, D. Caplan, and J. C. Marshall (eds.), *Neural models of language processes*. New York: Academic Press.

Marshall, J. C. (1984). Toward a rational taxonomy of the acquired dyslexias. In R. N. Malatesha and H. A. Whitaker (eds.), *Dyslexia: a global issue*. The Hague: Nijhoff.

Marshall, J. C. (1986). Description and interpretation of aphasic language disorder. *Neuropsychologia*, 24, 5–24.

Marshall, J. C. (1987). Routes and representations in the processing of written language. In E. Keller and M. Gopnik (eds.), *Motor and sensory processes of language*. Hillsdale, New Jersey: Lawrence Erlbaum Associates.

Marshall, J. C., and Newcombe, F. (1966). Syntactic and semantic errors in paralexia. *Neuropsychologia*, 4, 169–176.

Marshall, J. C., and Newcombe, F. (1973). Patterns of paralexia. *Journal of Psycholinguistic Research*, 2, 175–199.

Marshall, J. C., and Newcombe, F. (1988). Parasyndromes and paragrammatism. *Aphasiology*, 2, in press.

Marslen-Wilson, W. (1984). Function and process in spoken word recognition; a tutorial review. In H. Bouma and D. G. Bouwhuis (eds.), *Attention and performance X; control of language processes*. Hillsdale, New Jersey: Lawrence Erlbaum.

Marslen-Wilson, W. (1987). Functional parallelism in spoken word-recognition. *Cognition*, 25, 71–102.

Masterson, J. (1985). On how we read non-words: data from different populations. In K. E. Patterson, J. C. Marshall, and M. Coltheart (eds.), *Surface dyslexia: neuropsychological and cognitive analyses of phonological reading*. London: Lawrence Erlbaum.

McCarthy, R., and Warrington, E. K. (1984). A two route model of speech production; evidence from conduction aphasia. *Brain*, 107, 463–485.

McLelland, J. L., and Elman, J. L. (1985). Interactive processes in speech perception; the TRACE model. In J. L. McLelland and D. E. Rumelhart (eds.), *Parallel and distributed processing; explorations in the microstructure of cognition, volume 2*. Cambridge, Massachusetts: MIT Press.

Metz-Lutz, M-N., and Dahl, E. (1984). Analysis of word comprehension in a case of pure word deafness. *Brain and Language*, 23, 13–25.

Miceli, G., and Caramazza, A. (1988) Dissociation of inflectional and derivational morphology. *Brain and Language*, in press.

Miceli, G., Silveri, M. C., and Caramazza, A. (1987). The role of the phoneme-to-grapheme conversion system and the graphemic output buffer in writing. In M. Coltheart, G. Sartori, and R. Job (eds.), *The cognitive neuropsychology of language*. London: Lawrence Erlbaum Associates.

Michel, F. (1979). Préservation du langage écrit malgré un deficit majeur du langage oral (à propos d'un cas clinique). *Lyon Medicale*, 241, 141–149.

Michel, F., and Andreewsky, A. (1983). Deep dysphasia: an analog of deep dyslexia in the auditory modality. *Brain and Language*, 18, 212–223.

Monsell, S. (1985). Repetition and the lexicon. In A. W. Ellis (ed.), *Progress in the psychology of language, volume 2*. London: Lawrence Erlbaum.

Monsell, S. (1987a). On the relation between lexical input and output pathways. In D. A. Allport, D. MacKay, W. Prinz, and E. Scheerer (eds.), *Language perception and production; common processes in listening, speaking, reading and writing*. London: Academic Press.

Monsell, S. (1987b). Non-visual orthographic processing and the orthographic input lexicon. In M. Coltheart (ed.), *Attention and Performance XII*. London: Lawrence Erlbaum.

Morton, J. (1964). The effects of context on the visual duration threshold for words. *British Journal of Psychology*, 55, 165–180.

Morton, J. (1968). Grammar and computation in language behaviour. In J. C. Catford (ed.), *Studies in language and language behaviour*. C.R.L.L.B. Progress report no VI, University of Michigan.

Morton, J. (1969). The interaction of information in word recognition. *Psychological Review*, 76, 165–178.

Morton, J. (1970) A functional model for memory. In D. A. Norman (ed.), *Models for human memory*. New York: Academic Press.

Morton, J. (1979). Some experiments on facilitation of word and picture recognition and their relevance for the evolution of a theoretical position. In P. Kolers, M. Wrolstad, and H. Bouma (eds.), *Processing of visible language*. New York: Plenum.

Morton, J. (1980a). The logogen model and orthographic structure. In U. Frith (ed.), *Cognitive processes in spelling*. London: Academic Press.

Morton, J. (1980b). Two auditory parallels to deep dyslexia. In M. Coltheart, K. E. Patterson, and J. C. Marshall (eds.), *Deep dyslexia*. London: Routledge & Kegan Paul.

Morton, J. (1985). Naming. In S. K. Newman & R. Epstein (eds.), *Current perspectives in dysphasia*. Edinburgh: Churchill Livingstone.

Morton, J., and Patterson, K. E. (1980). A new attempt at an interpretation or an attempt at a new interpretation. In M. Coltheart, K. E. Patterson, and J. C. Marshall (eds.), *Deep dyslexia*. London: Routledge & Kegan Paul.

Newcombe, F., and Marshall, J. C. (1980). Transcoding and lexical stabilisation in deep dyslexia. In M. Coltheart, K. E. Patterson, and J. C. Marshall (eds.), *Deep dyslexia*. London: Routledge & Kegan Paul.

Newcombe, F., and Marshall, J. C. (1981). On the psycholinguistic classification of the acquired dyslexias. *Bulletin of the Orton Society*, 31, 29–46.

Newcombe, F., and Marshall, J. C. (1984). Task- and modality-specific aphasias. In F. C. Rose (ed.), *Advances in neurology, 42; progress in aphasiology*. New York: Raven Press.

Newcombe, F., and Marshall, J. C. (1985). Reading and writing by letter sounds. In, K. E. Patterson, J. C. Marshall, and M. Coltheart (eds.), *Surface dyslexia: neuropsychological and cognitive analyses of phonological reading*. London: Lawrence Erlbaum.

Nolan, K., and Caramazza, A. (1982). Modality independent impairments in processing in a deep dyslexia patient. *Brain and Language*, 16, 237–266.

Nolan, K., and Caramazza, A. (1983). An analysis of writing in a case of deep dyslexia. *Brain and Language*, 20, 305–328.

Parkin, A. J. (1982). Phonological recoding in lexical decision: effects of spelling-to-sound regularity depend on how regularity is defined. *Memory and Cognition*, 10, 43–53.

Pate, D. S., Saffran, E. M., and Schwartz, M. F. (1988). Specifying the locus of the impairment in conduction aphasia: a case study. *Language and Cognitive Processes*, 2,43–84.

Patterson, K. E. (1978). Phonemic dyslexia: errors of meaning and the meaning of errors. *Quarterly Journal of Experimental Psychology*, 30, 587–601.

Patterson, K. E. (1979). What is right with 'deep' dyslexic patients. *Brain and Language*, 8, 111–129.

Patterson, K. E. (1981). Neuropsychological approaches to the study of reading. *British Journal of Psychology*, 72, 151–174.

Patterson, K. E. (1982). The relationship between reading and phonological coding: further neuropsychological observations. In A. W. Ellis (ed.), *Normality and pathology in cognitive functions*. London: Lawrence Erlbaum.

Patterson. K. E. (1986). Lexical but non-semantic spelling? *Cognitive Neuropsychology*, 3, 341–367.

Patterson, K. E., and Besner, D. (1984). Is the right hemisphere literate? *Cognitive Neuropsychology*, 1, 315–341.

Patterson, K. E., and Morton, J. (1985). From orthography to phonology; an attempt at an old interpretation. In K. E. Patterson, J. C. Marshall, and M. Coltheart (eds.), *Surface dyslexia: neuropsychological and cognitive analyses of phonological reading*. London: Lawrence Erlbaum.

Patterson, K. E., and Coltheart, V. (1987). Phonological processes in reading: a tutorial review. In M. Coltheart (ed.), *Attention and performance XII*. London: Lawrence Erlbaum.

Patterson, K. E., Marshall, J. C., and Coltheart, M. (1985). *Surface dyslexia: neuropsychological and cognitive analyses of phonological reading*. London: Lawrence Erlbaum.

Patterson, K. E., Purell, C., and Morton, J. (1983). The facilitation of word retrieval in aphasia. In C. Code and D. J. Muller (eds.), *Aphasia therapy*. London: Edward Arnold.

Poeck, K., de Bleser, R., and von Keyserlingk, D. G. (1984). Computed tomography localisation of standard aphasic syndromes. In F. C. Rose (ed.), *Advances in neurology, 42; progress in aphasiology*. New York: Raven Press.

Rickard, S. (1986). Deep dyslexia. Unpublished PhD thesis, University of London.

Saffran, E. M. (1982). Neuropsychological approaches to the study of language. *British Journal of Psychology*, 73, 317–338.

Saffran, E., and Marin, O.S.M. (1977). Reading without phonology; evidence from aphasia. *Quarterly Journal of Experimental Psychology*, 29, 515–525.

Saffran, E. M., Bogyo, L. C., Schwartz, M. F., and Marin, O.S.M. (1980) Does deep dyslexia reflect right hemisphere reading? In M. Coltheart, K. E. Patterson, and J. C. Marshall (eds.) *Deep dyslexia*. London: Routledge and Kegan Paul.

Saffran, E. M., Marin, O.S.M., and Yeni-Komshian, G. H. (1976). An analysis of speech perception in word deafness. *Brain and Language*, 3, 209–228.

Scheerer, E. (1987). Visual word recognition in German. In D. A. Allport, D. MacKay, W. Prinz, and E. Scheerer (eds.), *Language perception and production; common processes in listening, speaking, reading and writing*. London: Academic Press.

Schwartz, M. F. (1984). What the classical aphasia categories can't do for us and why. *Brain and Language*, 21, 3–8.

Schwartz, M. F., Saffran, E. M., and Marin, O.S.M. (1980). Fractionating the reading process in dementia: evidence for word-specific print-to-sound associations. In M. Coltheart, K. E. Patterson and J. C. Marshall (eds.), *Deep dyslexia*. London: Routledge & Kegan Paul.

Seymour, P.H.K. (1979). *Human visual cognition*. London: Collier MacMillan.

Shallice, T. (1979a). The case study approach in neuropsychological research. *Journal of Clinical Neuropsychology*, 1, 183–211.

Shallice, T. (1979b) Neuropsychological research and the fractionation of memory systems. In L. J. Nilsson (ed.), *Perspectives on memory research*. Hillsdale, New Jersey: Lawrence Erlbaum Associates.

Shallice, T. (1987). Impairments of semantic processing: multiple dissociations. In M. Coltheart, R. Job, and G. Sartori (eds.), *The cognitive neuropsychology of language*. London: Lawrence Erlbaum.

Shallice, T. (1988). *From neuropsychology to mental structure*. Cambridge: Cambridge University Press.

Shallice, T., and McGill, J. (1978). The origins of mixed errors. In J. Requin (ed.), *Attention and performance VII*. Hillsdale, New Jersey: Lawrence Erlbaum Associates.

Shallice, T., and Vallar, G. (1989). Disorders of short term memory; a review of the syndrome. In T. Shallice and G. Vallar (eds.), *The neurological impairment of short term memory*. Cambridge: Cambridge University Press.

Shallice, T., and Warrington, E. K. (1975). Word recognition in a phonemic dyslexic patient. *Quarterly Journal of Experimental Psychology*, 27, 187–199.

Shallice, T., and Warrington, E. K. (1977). Auditory-verbal short term memory impairment and conduction aphasia. *Brain and Language*, 4, 479–491.

Shallice, T., and Warrington, E. K. (1980). Single and multiple component central dyslexic syndromes. In M. Coltheart, K. E. Patterson, and J. C. Marshall (eds.), *Deep dyslexia*. London: Routledge & Kegan Paul.

Shallice, T., McLeod, P., and Lewis, K. (1984). Isolating cognitive modules with the dual-task paradigm: are speech perception and production separate processes? *Quarterly Journal of Experimental Psychology*, 37A, 507–532.

Shallice, T., Warrington, E. K., and McCarthy, R. (1983). Reading without semantics. *Quarterly Journal of Experimental Psychology*, 35A, 111–138.

Shoumaker, R. D., Ajax, E. T., and Schenkenberg, T. (1977). Pure word deafness (auditory verbal agnosia). *Diseases of the Nervous System*, 38, 293–299.

Stemberger, J. P. (1985). An interactive activation model of language production. In A. W. Ellis (ed.), *Progress in the psychology of language, volume 1*. London: Lawrence Erlbaum Associates.

Symonds, C. (1953). Aphasia. *Journal of Neurology, Neurosurgery and Psychiatry*, 16, 1–16.

Thorndike, E. L., and Lorge, I. (1944). *The teacher's word book of 30,000 words*. New York: Teachers College, Columbia University.

Tyler, L. K. (1984). The structure of the initial cohort: evidence from gating. *Perception and Psychophysics*, 36, 417–427.

Tyler, L. K., and Wessels, J. (1983). Quantifying contextual contributions to word recognition processes. *Perception and Psychophysics*, 34, 409–420.

Underwood, G. (1977). Contextual facilitation from attended and unattended messages. *Journal of Verbal learning and Verbal Behaviour*, 16, 99–106.

Warren, R. M. (1970). Perceptual restoration of missing speech sounds. *Science*, 167, 392–393.

Warrington, E. K. (1975). The selective impairment of semantic memory. *Quarterly Journal of Experimental Psychology*, 27, 635–657.

Warrington, E. K. (1981). Concrete word dyslexia. *Brain*, 103, 99–112.

Warrington, E. K., and McKenna, P. (1983). *The Graded Naming Test*. London: NFER.

Warrington, E. K., and Shallice, T. (1984). Category-specific semantic impairment. *Brain*, 107, 829–854.

Wernicke, C. (1874). *Der aphasischer Symptomkomplex: eine psychologische Studie auf anatom-*

ischer Basis. Breslau: Cohn & Weigert. English translation by G. H. Eggert, 1977, in *Wernicke's works on aphasia: a sourcebook and review,* pp. 91–145. The Hague: Mouton.

Wernicke, C. (1885). Einige neuere Arbeiten über Aphasie. *Fortschritte der Medizin, 3,* 824. English translation by G. H. Eggert, 1977, in *Wernicke's works on aphasia: a sourcebook and review,* pp. 173–205. The Hague: Mouton.

Wernicke, C. (1906). Der aphasische Symptomenkomplex. *Die Deutsche Klinik am Eingange des 20 Jahrhunderts, 6,* 487. English translation by G. H. Eggert, 1977, in *Wernicke's works on aphasia: a sourcebook and review,* pp. 219–283. The Hague: Mouton.

Wernicke, C., and Friedlander, C. (1883). Ein Fall von Taubheit in Folge von doppelseitige Läsion des Schlafelappens. *Fortschritte der Medizin, 1.* English translation by G. H. Eggert, 1977, in *Wernicke's works on aphasia: a sourcebook and review,* pp. 164–172. The Hague: Mouton.

Wing, A. M., and Baddeley, A. B. (1980). Spelling errors in handwriting: a corpus and a distributional analysis. In U. Frith (ed.), *Cognitive processes in spelling.* London: Academic Press.

Winnick, W. A., and Daniel, S. A. (1970). Two kinds of response priming in tachistoscopic recognition. *Journal of Experimental Psychology, 84,* 74–81.

Yamadori, A., and Albert, M. L. (1973). Word category aphasia. *Cortex, 9,* 112–125.

Ziehl, F. (1896). Ueber einen Fall von Worttaubheit und das Lichtheim'sche Krankheitsbild der subcorticalen sensorischen Aphasie. *Deutsche Zeitschrift für Nervenheilkunde, 8,* 259–307.

Subject Index

Author Index